SILENT PARTNERS

Silent Partners

Human Subjects and Research Ethics

REBECCA DRESSER

OXFORD
UNIVERSITY PRESS

OXFORD
UNIVERSITY PRESS

Oxford University Press is a department of the University of Oxford. It furthers
the University's objective of excellence in research, scholarship, and education
by publishing worldwide. Oxford is a registered trade mark of Oxford University
Press in the UK and certain other countries.

Published in the United States of America by Oxford University Press
198 Madison Avenue, New York, NY 10016, United States of America.

© Oxford University Press 2017

Library of Congress Cataloging-in-Publication Data
Names: Dresser, Rebecca, author.
Title: Silent partners : human subjects and research ethics / Rebecca Dresser.
Description: Oxford ; New York : Oxford University Press, [2017] |
Includes index.
Identifiers: LCCN 2016012145 | ISBN 9780190459277 (alk. paper)
Subjects: | MESH: Ethics, Research | Human Experimentation—
ethics | Research Subjects | Bioethical Issues
Classification: LCC R853.H8 | NLM W 20.55.E7 | DDC 174.2/8—dc23 LC
record available at http://lccn.loc.gov/2016012145

Be approachable. Don't be judgmental. Hear what we say. Honestly listen to it.

—"What Women Who Use Drugs Have to Say about
Ethical Research," Kirsten Bell and Amy Salmon

When people ask, "Who watches the watchers?," why do they always leave out the possibility that the watched can watch as well?

—*War of the Encyclopaedists*,
Christopher Robinson and Gavin Kovite

CONTENTS

PREFACE

Ten years ago I faced a hard decision. I had just been diagnosed with advanced cancer. The doctor told me I had a 30–40 percent chance of surviving it. My choice was between two alternatives. One was a treatment regimen the hospital's tumor board, a group of cancer experts, had recommended for me. The other alternative was a clinical trial. If I chose the trial, I would be randomly assigned to receive one of two other treatment regimens the trial was evaluating.

The decision involved some clear trade-offs. The regimens being tested in the trial were less intensive than the regimen the tumor board had recommended. If I chose the tumor board's regimen, I would be treated with four chemotherapy drugs, including one the Food and Drug Administration had just approved for my kind of cancer. Then I would have several weeks of chemoradiation (combined chemotherapy and radiation therapy).

If I chose the trial, chance would determine my treatment. I would receive either three chemotherapy drugs plus chemoradiation or chemoradiation alone. Neither of the trial regimens offered the recently approved drug I would get if I took the tumor board's recommendation. Going into the trial would mean giving up the opportunity to receive that drug, as well as taking the chance that I would receive only chemoradiation. The trial would also require more meetings and paperwork, delaying the treatment I was desperate to start.

Frankly, I was terrified. The diagnosis had landed me in alien territory, and joining the trial would take me even further into the unknown. As a medical ethicist, I knew how important it was for patients like me to participate in trials. I knew that the treatment regimen the tumor board had recommended was based on information from trials that other patients had been willing to join. But the trial seemed less likely to save my life than the more intensive approach the tumor board had recommended.

I'm not a gambler by nature, and fear made me even more risk-averse than usual. Despite knowing—and appreciating—the research contributions my predecessors had made, I didn't follow their lead. I said no to the trial.

Looking back, I'm not sure I made the right decision. The treatment regimen I chose was successful and I am very happy to be alive. But the four-drug regimen was tough, with lots of side effects. It's quite possible that I would also have survived if I had chosen to join the trial. And given that the trial included fewer chemotherapy drugs, choosing the trial might have made my treatment less onerous.

I'm also a little ashamed that I said no to the trial. In refusing to become a research subject, I was putting my own desire to survive above the interests of future patients who might benefit from knowledge produced in the trial. Later I did agree to participate in some less demanding cancer research. But as a newly diagnosed and frightened cancer patient, I thought the treatment trial was asking too much of me.

This experience gave me a new understanding of what trial participation can look like from the perspective of a seriously ill patient.[1] Although I paid close attention to the doctor's factual description of my two options, fear, intuition, and the desire for self-preservation determined my ultimate choice. Despite being a research ethics "expert" as well as a longtime member of an institutional review board (a committee that considers the ethics of human studies), I had never realized what it would be like to deal with the kind of decision I faced.

Once my cancer treatment was over and I was back at work, I started reading about how other patients, as well as healthy volunteers, looked at their research experiences. I discovered that experienced subjects had a lot to say about what they had been through. To a reader like me, someone steeped in conventional thinking about research ethics, subjects presented the research process in a new and intriguing light. I thought that researchers and research ethicists should know more about what subjects were saying, so I began to work on this book.

Clinical trials like the one I considered are essential to advancing knowledge and improving human health. Biomedical researchers rely on human volunteers to test new ideas as well as potential medications and other treatment interventions. Human studies are conducted all over the world, and the demand for subjects is higher than ever.

As the biomedical research enterprise has grown, so has the field of research ethics. During the twentieth century it became clear that some subjects had been terribly mistreated in research—deceived, exposed to excessive risk, harmed in a variety of ways. Revelations of past research scandals led the

United States and other countries to develop regulations designed to protect human subjects. Institutional and government committees began reviewing study proposals to ensure that they met ethical standards and regulatory requirements for subject protection. In medical schools and universities, faculty and staff devoted considerable effort to addressing an array of ethical issues presented by different types of human studies.

Today one can find thousands of publications about human research ethics and regulation, as well as hundreds of government and professional reports on human subject issues. But few of those documents consider the views of people who have actually been research subjects. Instead, the views of professionals—researchers, ethicists, clinicians, and others—dominate the literature on human research ethics and policy.

This book is intended to address the imbalance. I believe that subjects' perspectives have been neglected in research ethics, and that the neglect has contributed to ongoing problems in research. People participating in research can contribute knowledge and ethical perspectives that are highly relevant to decisions about the acceptability of human studies. Indeed, it is a "very patronizing and paternalistic perspective" to assume that only researchers and other experts think about research ethics.[2]

In today's ethics and oversight system, decisions are made primarily by people who have never been research subjects. Their decisions are based on speculation about how subjects will experience study participation. For a variety of reasons, such speculative judgments can be inaccurate. Research experts and research subjects often occupy different social, cultural, educational, and economic positions. The same disparities can exist between subjects and members of the general public involved in research oversight. Moreover, as I learned, many people considering whether to participate in research are coping with serious illnesses and life circumstances that those involved in oversight have never personally faced. There can be large gaps between hypothetical and actual research experiences.

Rather than relying on speculation about the research participant experience, ethics and oversight ought to rely on what actual participants say about their experiences. Research ethics, as well as regulations intended to promote ethical conduct, should be based on evidence. Ethical and regulatory decisions should take into account participants' knowledge as well as their positions on ethical issues in research.

By considering actual subjects' perspectives, experts involved in the research enterprise can make more informed and ethical research decisions. People participating in research can supply facts about the experience that are otherwise overlooked or downplayed by those who have never been in the participants' position. Subjects' perspectives are "invaluable in reframing existing ethical issues in a more meaningful way, surfacing previously unidentified ethical issues, displaying divergent ethical priorities, re-evaluating the implications of research participation and restructuring researcher-participant relationships."[3] Trial participants are an "underutilized resource" whose "voice [is] largely ignored" in efforts to improve the informed consent process.[4] Decisions about acceptable research burdens should rely on information about subjects' actual concerns, instead of the concerns that reviewers assume subjects will have.[5]

Attention to subjects' perspectives makes sense from a broader policy standpoint too. Today's researchers face serious problems in enlisting and retaining a sufficient number of human subjects.[6] A significant number of clinical trials are discontinued, often because not enough people agree to participate. For example, one in five trials at four US National Cancer Institute Comprehensive Cancer Centers failed to enroll any subjects, and only fifty to sixty percent of trials at those centers met enrollment requirements.[7] Discontinued trials contribute nothing to the knowledge advances that justify the research enterprise. People enrolled in failed trials are also exposed to risk for no good reason. Failed trials consume finite resources as well. And researchers and clinicians waste their time and energy on activities that have no useful outcome.[8]

The failure to incorporate subjects' viewpoints into study planning and oversight decisions contributes to the current enrollment problems. Prospective subjects encounter "doctors and hospitals who have never considered how participation in trials feels to patients."[9] People will be reluctant to enroll in or complete studies that don't adequately address their concerns. They will be reluctant to participate in studies they consider overly burdensome or demanding. Information about subjects' perspectives is needed to determine when and why trials are likely to have difficulties recruiting and retaining subjects.

Research professionals have yet to recognize the distinct knowledge and ethical perspectives that experienced research subjects can bring to ethical and policy decisions about human research. Ethical and policy standards should take into account empirical and other information on subjects' views of the informed consent process, study burdens and benefits, and other ethical dimensions of research. Experienced subjects should also be part of the decision-making process. They should be members of research review committees, ethics and policy advisory groups, and groups advising researchers about specific human studies.

In the pages that follow, I describe what I have learned about subject perspectives and why this information is relevant to research ethics and policy. Although I focus on the views of experienced subjects, I also present information about prospective subjects' views. I use the terms "subject" and "participant" to refer to someone (other than researchers and their associates) involved in any stage of the research process, from study recruitment to completion. The terms "prospective subject" and "prospective participant" refer to someone responding to hypothetical research scenarios. The distinction between actual and prospective subjects is important, because people facing real research choices can have responses that differ from those of people imagining how they would respond to a hypothetical research situation.

The material in the book is meant to illustrate subjects' views. Although I refer to numerous narrative and empirical accounts, I don't claim to present a comprehensive review of the existing literature on subject perspectives. That literature presents a rich and complex picture of what research is like for subjects, and I could not possibly report everything in this volume. Also, as I note throughout the book, the existing literature doesn't always offer a representative indication of subjects' views on a given research question. More work will be needed to develop an adequate understanding of subject perspectives on a number of such questions.

Many thoughtful and generous people contributed to this book. For comments on parts of the manuscript, I thank Charlie Kurth, Stephen Lefrak, Nancy King, Norman Fost, Jill Fisher, Carl Elliott, Jim Lavery, Nancy Berlinger, Bruce

Jennings, Peter Joy, and anonymous reviewers for the *Journal of Law, Medicine & Ethics; Journal of Medical Ethics; Journal of Law and the Biosciences;* and Oxford University Press.

Presenting my ideas to various groups was immensely helpful too. I learned a great deal from participants in the Washington University Law School Faculty Workshop; Washington University Workshop on Politics, Ethics, and Society; Washington University Human Research Protection Office Ethics Series; Stanford University Law and Biosciences Workshop; University of Texas Law Review Symposium on Science Challenges for Law and Policy; Wake Forest University Law Review Symposium on Relationship-Centered Health Care; Public Responsibility in Medicine & Research Advancing Ethical Research Conference; and American Society for Bioethics and Humanities annual meetings. Phoebe Arde-Acquah provided extensive and valuable research assistance, finding many references I would otherwise have missed. I am grateful as well to Washington University Law School for financial support for the project.

Rebecca Dresser
St. Louis
January 2016

NOTES

1. For more about this experience and what it taught me, see Rebecca Dresser, "Volunteering for Research," in *Malignant: Medical Ethicists Confront Cancer*, ed. Rebecca Dresser (New York: Oxford University Press, 2012), 70–85.
2. See Susan Cox and Michael McDonald, "Ethics Is for Human Subjects Too: Participant Perspectives on Responsibility in

Health Research," *Social Science and Medicine* 98 (2013): 224–31.

3. Cox and McDonald, "Ethics Is for Human Subjects," 230.

4. Michele Eder et al., "Improving Informed Consent: Suggestions from Parents of Children with Leukemia," *Pediatrics* 119 (2007): e849–59.

5. Norma Morris and Brian Balmer, "Are You Sitting Comfortably? Perspectives of the Researchers and the Researched on 'Being Comfortable,'" *Accountability in Research* 13 (2006): 111–33.

6. Institute of Medicine, *Public Engagement and Clinical Trials: New Models and Disruptive Technologies: Workshop Summary* (2012). Retrieved March 25, 2015, from http://www.nap.edu/catalog/13237/public-engagement-and-clinical-trials-new-models-and-disruptive-technologies.

7. Gregory Curt and Bruce Chabner, "One in Five Cancer Trials Is Published: A Terrible Symptom—What's the Diagnosis?," *The Oncologist* 13 (2008): 923–24. See also Benjamin Kasenda et al., "Prevalence, Characteristics, and Publication of Discontinued Randomized Trials," *JAMA* 311 (2014): 1045–51; Ricki Carroll et al., "Motivations of Patients with Pulmonary Arterial Hypertension to Participate in Randomized Controlled Trials," *Clinical Trials* 9 (2012): 348–57. A review at the Oregon Health Sciences Center found that one million dollars was consumed in attempting to conduct trials that were later canceled or fell short of adequate enrollment. Peter Korn, "Clinical Trials Stymied as Patients Balk at 'Experiments,'" *Portland Tribune*, January 16, 2014. Retrieved April 15, 2015, from http://portlandtribune.com/pt/9-news/207447-63461-clinical-trials-stymied-as-patients-balk-at-experiments.

8. Alex London, Jonathan Kimmelman, and Marina Emborg, "Beyond Access vs. Protection in Trials of Innovative Therapies," *Science* 328 (2010): 829–30.

9. Korn, "Clinical Trials Stymied."

1

Subject Perspectives

The Missing Element in Research Ethics

■□■

THE ETHICAL PRINCIPLES AND REGULATIONS governing human subject research come largely from professionals— scientists, physicians, lawyers, and ethicists. Nearly everyone appointed to groups that develop and apply ethics standards is a professional. Although ordinary citizens are at times included in research ethics deliberations, they play a minor role. Most surprising—and disturbing—is the omission of people who know what it is like to be a research subject. Few people with direct experience as subjects have been involved in the creation and application of rules and guidelines for human subject research. Their exclusion has deprived the oversight system of morally relevant information.

History reveals a long-standing absence of experienced research subjects from ethical and policy deliberations. The Nuremberg Code, the first major document about human research ethics, is a set of principles created by physicians and

Parts of this chapter were previously published in "Research Subjects' Voices: The Missing Element in Research Ethics," *Anaesthesia and Intensive Care* 43 (2015): 297–99.

adopted by judges.[1] The World Medical Association, an organization of national medical societies, developed the Declaration of Helsinki, the most influential international statement on ethical standards for human research.[2] Scientists and officials at the National Institutes of Health (NIH) wrote the initial US human research guidelines. When public outcry over the infamous Tuskegee syphilis study moved Congress to address human research ethics, it established a national commission to develop more extensive research rules. Government officials appointed a group of professionals—lawyers, doctors, researchers, academics, and the president of a nonprofit organization—to that commission.[3]

Professionals addressing research ethics and oversight have experiences and interests that differ from those of research participants. Scientists and physicians emphasize the advances in knowledge and treatment that clinical research makes possible. Although some researchers serve as subjects during their student years, their experiences don't necessarily leave them with a long-standing sensitivity to subjects' interests and concerns. As investigators, their primary focus is on conducting efficient and successful human studies.

Researchers' professional roles shape their perceptions and judgments. "Researcher ethnocentrism"[4] can prevent researchers from seeing ethical problems with the design and conduct of human studies. It can also lead them to resist the delays and impediments that can accompany efforts to promote subjects' autonomy and well-being. Although physicians have a duty to promote the best interests of their patients, including those considering participating in studies, many physicians are also directly or indirectly involved in the research enterprise. Physicians strongly committed to research objectives may overlook or downplay the risks and other challenges that patient-subjects encounter in clinical trials.[5]

Professionals from other fields also have research perspectives that differ from those of research subjects. Experts from fields like bioethics and law typically lack experience as research subjects. Many are employees of academic institutions with major biomedical research programs. Like researchers and physicians, they have competing interests— allegiance to colleagues, institutions, and medical progress competes with allegiance to subject protection. Professionals working for patient advocacy organizations like the March of Dimes, Juvenile Diabetes Association, and American Cancer Society tend to be most interested in advancing research that will contribute to medical improvements for their constituents.

Although professionals have dominated activities relating to research ethics and policy, the general public has not been completely left out. National and other research ethics groups sometimes include public representatives, and US regulations require institutional review boards (IRBs), the committees that review the ethics of human research proposals, to include "at least one member who is not otherwise affiliated with the institution."[6] But public representatives don't necessarily bring the perspective of research participants to the table. Public members of these groups are not required to have had experience as research subjects, nor are they assigned to represent subjects' interests.[7] Indeed, members of the general public have strong interests in promoting research that could lead to healthcare improvements for themselves and their loved ones. As a result, public representatives may assign a higher value to research advances than to subjects' interests and concerns.

In their research ethics work, most professionals and members of the general public strive to safeguard subjects' interests. Yet these professionals and public representatives often lack the personal experience that would enhance their ability to speak for subjects. People who have never been in the research subject's position are often unaware of pressures, concerns, and other on-the-ground realities that subjects encounter. Although many members of research teams do have on-the-ground experience with the research process, they see studies through a particular lens, one that may distort or exclude aspects of participants' experiences. Professionals and public representatives tend to assume they are representing subjects' perspectives without testing the validity of their assumptions.[8]

The failure to solicit meaningful input from experienced research subjects in ethics deliberations, policy formation, and oversight is at odds with the egalitarian vision of human research. In considering the morality of human research, influential thinkers like Paul Ramsey and Jay Katz used terms like "co-adventurers," "joint adventurers," and "partnership" to describe the ideal relationship between investigators and subjects.[9] Philosopher Hans Jonas envisioned a similar model in which study investigators and volunteers are equally committed to the research cause.[10] Much of the contemporary rhetoric about clinical research also refers to researchers and subjects as equal contributors to the research endeavor.[11] Consistent with this thinking, today's study volunteers are often referred to as "research participants" instead of "research subjects"—a move intended to put subjects and investigators on an equal footing.[12]

Though the prevailing rhetoric presents study participants as equal partners in research, the reality is quite different. Professionals and a few public representatives evaluate the morality of research without material input from research subjects. Although those in charge of this process attempt to incorporate subjects' perspectives, they typically rely on assumptions rather than actual subject input. To date, subjects' perceptions and preferences have had little impact on the ethical standards and policies governing human research.

The experiences and viewpoints of research subjects merit much more attention than they have received. As Katz warned, ethical codes "divorced from the realities of human interaction ... invite judicious or injudicious neglect."[13] Codes and policies devised by professionals are in danger of suffering from this neglect. For example, there is a large gap between the ethical and policy requirements for informed consent to research and the actual understanding of many participants.[14] Although experts have developed defensible consent standards, the standards have proven difficult to put into practice.

Moreover, personal experience as a study subject produces knowledge relevant to research ethics and policy. Many people, including researchers and individuals involved in research oversight, have described how experience as a subject opened their eyes to previously unappreciated features of study participation.[15] As I say in the preface, the idea for this book arose from my own firsthand experiences as a cancer patient considering participation in a clinical trial.[16]

In addition to the researchers, physicians, and ethicists who have described personal experiences as research subjects,[17] many other people have written about their experiences as subjects or have told their stories to journalists and scholars.[18] This literature remains a largely untapped resource for developing a more subject-centered account of research ethics. Empirical studies are another source of information about subjects' perspectives on research. Such studies collect data on subjects' experiences with research as well as their views on specific topics, such as payment for participation and the effectiveness of various approaches to protecting subjects from harm.[19] This empirical literature offers a wealth of information relevant to research ethics and policy.

This book moves research subject perspectives to the forefront. I analyze a variety of ethical and regulatory matters in light of what subjects and potential subjects say about research. I consider personal accounts from individuals who completed participation in research trials and from those who dropped out of trials or declined participation after considering enrollment. I discuss how this material relates to a range of activities relevant to human research ethics, including the work of government and professional groups addressing the ethical dimensions of different kinds of research as well as the work of national and institutional groups evaluating the ethics of specific research proposals.

OVERLOOKING SUBJECTS: A HISTORY

In examining the role of subjects in research ethics deliberations, I return to a question raised decades ago by medical ethicist Robert Veatch. In a 1975 article, Veatch described the emergence of ethics review at the NIH.[20] Initially, researchers' scientific colleagues were responsible for evaluating the ethics of proposed studies. Later, members of Congress and others pressed NIH officials to include a wider array of professionals, such as lawyers, theologians, and philosophers, in research ethics review.[21] These critics thought that an interdisciplinary group of professionals was needed to ensure that publicly funded research was conducted in an ethical manner.

But there were also calls for an even broader approach. One early supporter of such an approach was James Shannon, the director of NIH from 1955 to 1968. In 1964, NIH advisers recommended that Shannon appoint a group of professionals to develop ethical principles for human research. But Shannon was dissatisfied with this recommendation. In a response to the advisers, he wrote, "To win general acceptance within not only the medical community but also our society at large," the ethical principles "should probably emerge from a group which includes representatives of the whole ethical, moral, and legal interests of society."[22] Veatch characterized Shannon's statement as a "profound insight [that] projected the evolution of the layperson's role in experimentation review over the next decade up to the present."[23]

A few years after Shannon's statement, officials began to list "community acceptance" as an important element of ethics review. At one point in the 1970s, draft NIH regulations required review boards to have members "competent to represent the community from which the subject population is drawn."[24] But later drafts omitted this language, and the final regulations, issued in 1981, required only that review boards have at least one member with no personal or financial connection to the research institution. Similarly, today's IRB regulations make no reference to representation of the subject population, noting only that IRBs should include individuals with "sensitivity to such issues as community attitudes."[25]

As Veatch saw it, this history exposed a central question for those designing and running a system for reviewing research ethics: Should judgments about research ethics be made by professionals alone or by representatives of the wider community as well? Veatch acknowledged that professionals have access to facts that are relevant to ethical judgments, such as information about research procedures, research risks, and existing knowledge about a research area. But Veatch argued that experts are incapable of making certain "reasonable person" judgments that are essential to ethical review. To meet standards of informed consent, for example, reviewers must determine what a reasonable person would want to know about a study. Reasonable-person judgments are also essential to determining whether risks to subjects are justified by the importance of the knowledge a study is expected to generate.

Reasonable-person judgments are properly made by "peers of the subjects," Veatch contended, not by professionals. Ordinary people are best situated to determine what prospective subjects would want to know about a study before enrolling. And because professionals as a class place a high value on advancing knowledge, he wrote, they usually assign great weight to the benefits of research. This value judgment can lead professionals to see research risks as justified when laypersons might have a different view. Veatch believed that ordinary citizens can best represent the general community in determining whether research risks are reasonable in light of the benefits a study is expected to produce.

Veatch made a valuable contribution in highlighting the differences between professional and citizen review, but he failed to recognize that members of the general public are not full "peers of the subject." Certainly members of the general public have a legitimate role in ethical decision-making about human research, but a truly representative group would also include members with actual experience as study subjects. Veatch's larger point still stands, however: professionals have disproportionate power over decisions about research ethics.

In establishing government requirements for research ethics review, officials chose to rely primarily on professionals to evaluate proposed human studies. The regulatory requirements for public involvement are minimal. But Shannon's community acceptance ideal is unlikely to be achieved with the inclusion of only a few laypersons in research ethics activities. And an even bigger policy problem is the absence of a requirement to include individuals who have served as research subjects among those reviewing the ethics of human research.

SUPPORT FOR SUBJECT INCLUSION

In the decades after Veatch's article, others have pressed for increased diversity in deliberations about ethics and policy. Scholars, researchers, clinicians, and public officials have endorsed ideas and programs that provide support for including experienced research subjects in ethical decision-making. Work in deliberative democracy, feminist epistemology, narrative medicine, and participatory research supplies rationales for integrating subject perspectives into the decision-making process.

Deliberative democracy is a concept that promotes public participation in policymaking. Although writers examining deliberative democracy focus on politics and government policy, they also consider other forms of collective decision-making. Deliberative democracy supports including subjects in research ethics decision-making. Two leading theorists, Amy Gutmann and Dennis Thompson, believe that deliberative democracy is particularly well suited to forums involving bioethics, such as IRBs and ethics advisory groups.[26]

Iris Marion Young's work on deliberative democracy is particularly relevant to the research situation. Young sees inclusion as a way to promote legitimacy, justice, and wisdom in deliberations about social issues. She believes that people "expected to abide by rules or adjust their actions" based on the outcome of a deliberative process ought to have a voice in that process.[27] Allowing all affected persons to be represented demonstrates moral respect for those persons and produces more just resolutions as well. When different groups are represented in deliberation, Young asserts, the self-interested claims of one group are likely to be scrutinized and challenged by other participants. Inclusion thus reduces the chance that deliberation will produce biased outcomes.

Young contends that inclusion also leads to more informed decisions. No single individual or group is aware of every fact relevant to resolving a social issue. Factors like culture, gender, class, and social position affect what a person knows about an issue. Deliberation that solicits input from people with different perspectives on an issue "produces a collective social wisdom not available from any one position," Young writes.[28]

Achieving the goals of inclusion requires the presence of people with different perspectives. In debates over social issues, Young writes, it is common for people to assume "that they know what it is like for others, or that they can put themselves in the place of the others, or that they are just like the others."[29] But such assumptions can generate misguided deliberative outcomes, Young warns. This is just what can happen when experienced subjects are absent from research ethics decision-making.

Young and other deliberative democracy theorists are beginning to have an impact on research practices. Some ethicists and researchers have created deliberative forums to address topics like human tissue research and surrogate consent to research.[30] Although these forums usually involve members of the general public, a few focus on members of populations likely to be approached about specific types of research participation. For example, a project on surrogate consent to research solicited input from people who were caregivers or primary decision-makers for people with dementia.[31] In later parts of this book, I discuss deliberative democratic approaches to specific research questions, such as whether results of genetic research should be returned to subjects. Projects like these can serve as models for including individuals with experience as subjects in research ethics deliberations.

Feminist epistemology theory and a related philosophical approach called standpoint theory also supply support for including subjects in research ethics decision-making. These two philosophical approaches emphasize how personal experience affects the production of knowledge. They challenge conventional notions of objectivity, contending instead that everyone, including scientists and other experts, is a "situated knower."[32] Each knower's thinking is influenced by that person's individual and social circumstances. Everyone brings particular background assumptions to the table, bias is inevitable, and no one is truly objective.

Scholars in feminist epistemology and standpoint theory examine how biology, psychology, philosophy, and other fields have been affected by the exclusion of women and other groups. These scholars believe that traditional forms of knowledge production have generated biased findings and conclusions. Higher-quality theory and policy come, they say, when knowledge production involves an array of people with diverse perspectives, values, and interests.[33]

Like deliberative democracy, feminist epistemology and standpoint theory support the inclusion of experienced subjects in deliberations about research ethics, in that a group with distinct insights has traditionally been absent from the production and application of research ethics knowledge. The reasoning underlying these approaches suggests that the failure to include experienced subjects has produced deficient policies and practices governing human subject research.

Narrative medicine is another source of support for subject inclusion. Narrative medicine promotes the use of personal stories to understand illness, suffering, and the medical response to these conditions. Narratives have become popular because first-person accounts from patients, their families, and clinicians offer insights that are inaccessible through more conventional forms of medical inquiry.[34] Storytellers give readers and listeners a detailed and nuanced picture of what it is like to live with disease, cope with invasive and burdensome treatments, and confront mortality. Personal narratives can be particularly valuable in medical ethics, because they provide rich case examples, provoke moral reflection, and inform ethical judgments.[35]

So far, narrative medicine has emphasized ways in which first-person accounts can enhance clinical education and practice. But narrative approaches can be just as enlightening in the research context. Personal accounts from experienced subjects reveal whether central ethical concepts like informed consent and risk minimization are meaningfully applied in the real world. Such accounts also draw attention to unexposed features of human research that require ethical and policy responses.[36] Subjects' narratives offer researchers and research ethicists a resource for understanding what qualifies as ethical human research.

New models of health research supply yet another basis for subject inclusion. Participatory research and other forms of community-engaged research respond to dissatisfaction with the traditional research hierarchy, in which studies are "done on participants rather than by or for them."[37] Such initiatives give members of study populations opportunities to collaborate in creating, conducting, and interpreting findings from specific studies.[38] These new models arose first in international development projects and public health research, but they are now being adopted in medical research as well.[39]

In participatory and community-engaged research, people from community and illness groups are seen as experts whose knowledge can enhance the quality and value of research. For example, patients and community members know about the types of studies that their peers need most. They also know about strategies that will be acceptable and effective in recruiting subjects, as well as ways to connect research findings to actual health improvements.[40]

Supporters of these nontraditional research models often cite ethical justifications for collaborating with patients and community members. They say that collaborative methods demonstrate respect for people who participate in studies as well as for those affected by study outcomes. Such methods can also correct the power imbalances that have given rise to unjust research burdens on disadvantaged groups.[41] By collaborating with members of a subject population, researchers can discover how best to explain studies to potential participants, thus promoting autonomous decisions about study enrollment. Collaboration also increases the likelihood that study subjects and their peers will benefit from their research contributions.[42]

THEMES AND CHALLENGES

Although researchers increasingly recognize, or at least accept, the calls for including subjects and prospective subjects in planning, conducting, and interpreting human studies, ethicists lag behind. Not many groups addressing research ethics have invited ordinary citizens, much less experienced study participants, to the table. Few ethics experts seem to regard actual and prospective subjects as essential contributors to ethical judgments about human research. For example, the voices of experienced subjects are rarely heard in debates over topics like the effectiveness of IRBs and the proper consent requirements for research comparing current medical practices.[43] Ethicists and advisory groups take positions on matters like these without consulting the people who will be most affected by policy decisions.

Ethical standards and regulatory rules should be informed by the perceptions and judgments of individuals who serve as research subjects. Deliberative research forums and participatory research are a beginning, but much more is needed. Meaningful change will require softening the traditional boundary between research experts and research subjects.[44] Research professionals accustomed to control must see subjects as experts with distinct and valuable contributions to make to research evaluation and oversight. Subjects are the only people who know what it is like to confront complicated consent forms and discussions and make important personal decisions based on them. Subjects are also the only people to bear the actual burdens and inconveniences of study participation, and to juggle the responsibilities of participation with the demands of everyday life. Research decisions that rely on subject input will be ethically and practically superior to those that rely on speculation about such matters.

In the chapters that follow, I show how information about subjects' perspectives supplements and challenges conventional positions on human research ethics. I also consider how rules and practices governing human research could be revised to reflect study participants' views and insights. To explore the world of research subjects, I turn to a variety of sources: empirical research on subjects' perceptions and viewpoints; subjects' personal accounts of participation; and media stories reporting on subjects' experiences.

Chapter 2, "Personal Knowledge and Study Participation," examines the educational value of becoming a research subject. Scientists in earlier times considered self-experimentation an essential component of their work. They thought that exposing themselves to untested interventions was the most ethical way to gauge the human response to those interventions. The practice was also educational, for it produced information that helped researchers plan subsequent human studies. Self-experimentation was eventually replaced by more sophisticated scientific methods and comprehensive ethical codes governing human research. But it is time to bring back the practice of self-experimentation, albeit in modified form. Serving as a study subject can be a valuable form of education for people who conduct and review proposals for human research.

Chapter 3, "The Everyday Ethics of Human Research," describes subjects' views on their research experiences. Subjects have their own opinions about research ethics. For example, a study staff's kind or rude behavior strongly influences whether subjects feel respected in the research process. Subjects also describe burdens of study participation that researchers and other outsiders don't always recognize. People deciding whether to allow a family member with dementia to participate in research tend to be more concerned about protecting the relative's current welfare than about promoting his or her previous values. Findings like these show what people with personal research experience can contribute to the work of research ethics review committees, study teams designing and conducting research, and groups developing ethical and regulatory policies on specific research questions.

Chapter 4, "The Hidden World of Subjects: Rule Breaking in Clinical Trials," looks at subjects' concealed misbehavior in research. When their personal interests conflict with the demands of participation, some subjects put their own interests first. They don't follow study requirements and try to hide this from researchers. In rejecting the restrictions research imposes, subjects diminish the value of research results. They create risks to themselves and others; they also disregard ethical responsibilities to adhere to research agreements and tell the truth. At the same time, rule-breaking subjects expose ethical problems in the design and conduct of clinical trials. Features of the research environment create fertile ground for concealed rule breaking. Intensified policing and guidance are two common strategies for reducing subject misbehavior, but collaborative reforms are more consistent with the partnership model of clinical research.

Chapter 5, "Participants as Partners in Genetic Research," focuses on subject-centered developments in genetic research. Modern genetic research requires scientists to collect, store, and study DNA samples and health information from thousands of people. In the past, researchers have been allowed to use DNA samples and information without consent. Researchers have not been required to explain study results to subjects, nor to compensate people who contribute samples and health information to genetic studies. Experts developed these practices without input from the people whose contributions are essential to the genetic research enterprise. A growing amount of evidence shows that many research subjects and prospective subjects disagree with these traditional approaches. For ethical and practical reasons, subjects should have a greater role in determining how genetic research is conducted.

Chapter 6, "Terminally Ill Patients and the 'Right to Try' Experimental Drugs," addresses access to unapproved drugs. Some terminally ill patients enroll in research as a way to gain access to experimental drugs. Other patients want to try the drugs without enrolling in research. The US Food and Drug Administration permits patients to do so under certain circumstances, but critics say the government rules are too restrictive. "Right to try" advocates campaign for laws permitting more liberal access, telling heart-wrenching stories about patients desperate to obtain experimental drugs. But the picture they present is one-sided. Stories conveying the harm that can come from access to these drugs belong in the debate too.

Chapter 7, "Embedded Ethics in Developing-Country Research" considers subject inclusion in multinational studies. Many studies are initiated and financed by wealthy countries but conducted in low-income countries. Community engagement and participatory research have a long history in developing-country research. Over the years, there has been impressive progress in including experienced subjects and other community members in research activities. This progress is due in part to the contributions of social scientists examining and evaluating ways to involve subjects and other community residents in research decisions. The practice of "embedded ethics" should be applied in domestic research as well.

Chapter 8, "Research Subjects as Literary Subjects," turns to literature for insights on what it is like to be a research subject. Many creative writers look at research through the eyes of research subjects. They apply imagination and literary skills to bring the research world to life. Fictional accounts like *White Noise* and *The Normals* (novels about healthy volunteers in phase 1 drug studies), "Escape from Spiderhead" (a short story about prison research), and *We Are Not Ourselves* (a novel describing participation in an Alzheimer's drug study) illuminate ethical dimensions of the human subject experience. Creative writers portray research experiences in fresh and vivid ways, and research professionals can learn from them.

Chapter 9, "How to Hear Subjects" makes the case for including experienced subjects in a variety of activities relating to research ethics and policy. People with direct experience as research subjects should be involved in research review as well as in community-engaged and patient-centered research efforts. Experienced subjects should also be included in advisory groups considering ethical and policy topics like informed consent and comparative-effectiveness research. Achieving subject inclusion will require attention to matters such as selection criteria and training for subjects participating in ethics and policy activities. But the inclusion challenges should not be exaggerated; adding subjects to research ethics activities is a manageable step toward an improved research enterprise.

Although I believe that subject inclusion is achievable, I don't mean to suggest it will be easy. As Young concedes, inclusion can complicate and impede consensus building in deliberative forums.[45] Bringing to the surface unrecognized and underappreciated aspects of human research could lead to longer and less harmonious deliberations for IRBs and other ethics advisory groups. Young also warns that the pure presence of a previously excluded group is insufficient to create genuine inclusion. People newly admitted to deliberative forums "sometimes find that those still more powerful in the process exercise, often unconsciously, a new form of exclusion: others ignore or dismiss or patronize their statements and expressions."[46] What Young refers to as "internal exclusion" is something that laypersons often experience when they are asked to participate in activities dominated by research professionals.[47] Later chapters consider these and other inclusion challenges as they arise in specific research contexts.

The knowledge gained through personal research experience is not the only relevant factor in determining either the characteristics of an ethical study or the general ethical and regulatory principles governing human research. Professional knowledge belongs in the mix as well. Similarly, subjects' preferences and interests should not completely control decisions about research ethics and policy. Those decisions must take into account the interests of future patients, researchers, and the broader society too. But subjects' personal perspectives on research have been neglected for too long. Progress in research ethics and oversight requires deeper engagement with people who have direct experience as human subjects.

NOTES

1. See Jonathan Moreno, *Undue Risk: Secret State Experiments on Humans* (New York: W. H. Freeman, 2000).
2. Richard Ashcroft, "The Declaration of Helsinki," in *The Oxford Textbook of Clinical Research Ethics*, ed. Ezekiel Emanuel et al. (New York: Oxford University Press, 2008), 141–48.
3. The National Commission for the Protection of Human Subjects in Biomedical and Behavioral Research issued a series of reports and recommendations that became the basis of US regulations governing human research. See Tom Beauchamp, "The Belmont Report," in *The Oxford Textbook of Clinical Research Ethics*, ed. Ezekiel Emanuel et al. (New York: Oxford University Press, 2008), 149–55.
4. John Lynch, "'Through a Glass Darkly': Researcher Ethnocentrism and the Demonization of Research Participants," *American Journal of Bioethics*, 11, no. 4 (2011): 22–23.
5. Jay Katz, "The Regulation of Human Research—Reflections and Proposals," *Clinical Research* 21 (1973): 785–91; Samuel Hellman and Deborah Hellman, "Of Mice but Not Men: Problems of the Randomized Clinical Trial," *New England Journal of Medicine* 324 (1991): 1585–89.
6. "Federal Policy for the Protection of Human Subjects," 56 *Fed. Reg.* 28,015 (June 18, 1991).
7. Rebecca Dresser, *When Science Offers Salvation: Patient Advocacy and Research Ethics* (New York: Oxford University Press, 2001), 109–28.

8. See Laura Stark, *Behind Closed Doors: IRBs and the Making of Ethical Research* (Chicago: University of Chicago Press, 2012), 13–15, 21–39.
9. See Paul Ramsey, *The Patient as Person: Explorations in Medical Ethics* (New Haven: Yale University Press, 1970), 5–7; Katz, "Regulation of Human Research," 787. Although Katz endorsed the partnership model on moral grounds, he also recognized that "physician-investigators do not consider . . . patient-subjects as equal partners in the decision-making process." Jay Katz, "Human Experimentation and Human Rights," *St. Louis University Law Review* 38 (1993): 7–54, 14.
10. Hans Jonas, "Philosophical Reflections on Experimenting with Human Subjects," *Daedalus*, 98, no. 2 (1969): 219–47, 236.
11. For example, G. Owen Schaefer, Ezekiel Emanuel, and Alan Wertheimer, "The Obligation to Participate in Research," *Journal of the American Medical Association* 302, no. 1 (2009): 67–72, 68; Ezekiel Emanuel, David Wendler, and Christine Grady, "What Makes Clinical Research Ethical?," *Journal of the American Medical Association* 283 (2000): 2701–11.
12. Emanuel, Wendler, and Grady, "What Makes Clinical Research Ethical?," 2707. I use the terms *subject* and *participant* interchangeably because I believe that *subject* is still an accurate descriptor. Individuals can decide whether to participate in studies, but they typically have little say over anything else related to study participation.
13. Jay Katz, "The Education of the Physician-Investigator," *Daedalus* 98, no. 2 (1969): 480–501, 483.
14. James Flory, David Wendler, and Ezekiel Emanuel, "Empirical Issues in Informed Consent for Research," in *The Oxford Textbook of Clinical Research Ethics*, ed. Ezekiel Emanuel et al. (New York: Oxford University Press, 2008), 645–60.
15. Alan Wertheimer, "Non-completion and Informed Consent," *Journal of Medical Ethics* 40 (2014): 127–30; Jack Coulehan, "My Battle against Gonorrhea," *Annals of Internal Medicine* 155 (2011): 198–200; Public Responsibility in Medicine & Research, "In Their Own Voices: A Discussion with Research

Subjects Who Also Work in the Field of Subject Protection," December 12, 2010. Retrieved March 6, 2015, from https://www.conferencepassport.com/index.asp.

16. Rebecca Dresser, "Volunteering for Research," in *Malignant: Medical Ethicists Confront Cancer*, ed. Rebecca Dresser (New York: Oxford University Press, 2012), 70–85.

17. Wertheimer, "Non-completion and Informed Consent"; Coulehan, "My Battle against Gonorrhea."

18. See, for example, Roberto Abadie, *The Professional Guinea Pig: Big Pharma and the Risky World of Human Subjects* (Durham, NC: Duke University Press, 2010); Jill Fisher, *Medical Research for Hire: The Political Economy of Pharmaceutical Clinical Trials* (New Brunswick, NJ: Rutgers University Press, 2009); Robert Helms, ed., *Guinea Pig Zero: An Anthology of the Journal for Human Research Subjects* (New Orleans: Garrett County Press, 2002); Martin Patriquin, "Inside the Human Guinea Pig Capital of North America," *MacLean's* 122, no. 33 (2009); Barbara Solow, "The Secret Lives of Guinea Pigs," *Independent Weekly*, February 9, 2000; Laurie P. Cohen, "Stuck for Money: To Screen New Drugs for Safety, Lilly Pays Homeless Alcoholics," *Wall Street Journal*, November 14, 1996; Josh McHugh, "Drug Test Cowboys: The Secret World of Pharmaceutical Trial Subjects," *Wired*, April 24, 2007. Retrieved February 20, 2015, from http://www.wired.com/wired/archive/15.05/feat_drugtest.html.

19. See Leanne Stunkel and Christine Grady, "More than the Money: A Review of the Literature Examining Healthy Volunteer Motivations," *Contemporary Clinical Trials* 32 (2011): 342–52; R. Hermann et al., "Adverse Events and Discomfort in Studies on Healthy Subjects: The Volunteer's Perspective," *European Journal of Clinical Pharmacology* 53 (1997): 207–14.

20. Robert Veatch, "Human Experimentation Committees: Professional or Representative?," *Hastings Center Report* 5, no. 5 (1975): 31–40.

21. This evolution is described in detail in Stark, *Behind Closed Doors*, 75–158.

22. Mark Frankel, "The Development of Policy Guidelines Governing Human Experimentation in the United States," *Ethics in Science and Medicine* 2, no. 5 (1975): 43–59, 51. In a 1965 presentation to an NIH oversight group, Shannon challenged the traditional view that laypersons "were not qualified to pass judgment on the ethical aspects of medical research." Charles McCarthy, "The Origins and Policies That Govern Institutional Review Boards," in *The Oxford Textbook of Clinical Research Ethics* ed. Ezekiel Emanuel et al. (New York: Oxford University Press, 2008), 541–51, 542.

23. Veatch, "Human Experimentation Committees," 34.

24. Ibid.

25. "Federal Policy for the Protection of Human Subjects," 28,015.

26. Amy Gutmann and Dennis Thompson, "Deliberating about Bioethics," *Hastings Center Report* 27, no. 3 (1997): 38–41. Govind Persad also argues that deliberative democracy provides support for including research subjects in ethics review. See Govind Persad, "Democratic Deliberation and the Ethical Review of Human Subject Research," in *Human Subjects Research Regulation: Perspectives on the Future*, ed. I. Glenn Cohen and Holly Fernandez Lynch (Cambridge, MA: MIT Press, 2014), 169–84.

27. Iris Marion Young, *Inclusion and Democracy* (Oxford: Oxford University Press, 2000), 23.

28. Ibid., 76.

29. Ibid., 77.

30. Kieran O'Doherty, Alice Hawkins, and Michael Burgess, "Involving Citizens in the Ethics of Biobank Research: Informing Institutional Policy through Structured Public Deliberation," *Social Science and Medicine* 75 (2012): 1604–11; Raymond De Vries, Aimee Stanczyk, Ian Wall et al., "Assessing the Quality of Democratic Deliberation: A Case Study of Public Deliberation on the Ethics of Surrogate Consent for Research," *Social Science and Medicine* 70 (2010): 1896–903; Scott Kim, Ian Wall, and Aimee Stanczyk, "Assessing the Public's Views in Research Ethics Controversies: Deliberative Democracy and Bioethics as Natural Allies," *Journal of*

Empirical Research on Human Research Ethics 4, no. 4 (2009): 3–16.

31. De Vries et al., "Assessing the Quality," 1897.
32. Elizabeth Anderson, "Feminist Epistemology and Philosophy of Science," in *The Stanford Encyclopedia of Philosophy* (2011). Retrieved July 5, 2013, from http://plato.stanford.edu/entries/feminism-epistemology/.
33. Anderson, "Feminist Epistemology."
34. Rita Charon, "Narrative Medicine: A Model for Empathy, Reflection, Profession, and Trust," *Journal of the American Medical Association* 286 (2001): 1897–902.
35. Ann Hudson Jones, "Narrative in Medical Ethics," *BMJ* 318 (1999): 253–56.
36. Wertheimer, "Non-completion and Informed Consent."
37. Andrea Cornwell, "Toward Participatory Practice: Participatory Rural Appraisal (PRA) and the Participatory Process," in *Participatory Research in Health: Issues and Experiences*, ed. Korrie de Koning and Marion Martin (Atlantic Highlands, NJ: Zed Books, 1996), 94.
38. Dan O'Connor, "The Apomediated World: Regulating Research When Research Has Changed," *Journal of Law, Medicine & Ethics* 41 (2013): 470–83; Sharon Terry and Patrick Terry, "Power to the People: Participant Ownership of Clinical Trial Data," *Science Translational Medicine* 3 (2011): 1–4; Effy Vayena et al., "Research Led by Participants: A New Social Contract for a New Kind of Research," *Journal of Medical Ethics*. Published online first: April 13, 2015, doi:10.1136/medethics-2015-102663.
39. Ethan Basch, "Toward Patient-Centered Drug Development in Oncology," *New England Journal of Medicine* 369 (2013): 397–400; Loretta Jones and Kenneth Wells, "Strategies for Academic and Clinician Engagement in Community-Participatory Partnered Research," *Journal of the American Medical Association* 297 (2007): 407–10.
40. Mary Tinetti and Ethan Basch, "Patients' Responsibility to Participate in Decision Making and Research," *Journal of the American Medical Association* 309 (2013): 2331–32; Dresser, *When Science Offers Salvation*, 23–29.

41. Sara Goering, Suzanne Holland, and Kelly Fryer-Edwards, "Transforming Genetic Research Practices with Marginalized Communities: A Case for Responsive Justice," *Hastings Center Report* 38, no. 2 (2008): 43–53.
42. Ibid.
43. For discussion of the IRB controversy, see Steven Joffe, "Revolution or Reform in Human Subjects Research Oversight," *Journal of Law, Medicine & Ethics* 40 (2012): 922–29; Alex John London, "A Non-paternalistic Model of Research Ethics Oversight: Assessing the Benefits of Prospective Review," *Journal of Law, Medicine & Ethics* 40 (2012): 930–44. For discussion of the informed consent question, see Emily Anderson and Stephanie Solomon, "Community Engagement: Critical to Continued Public Trust in Research," *American Journal of Bioethics* 13, no. 12 (2013): 44–46; "Ethical Oversight of Learning Health Care Systems," special supplement, *Hastings Center Report* 43, no. 1 (2013); Robert Truog, Walter Robinson, Adrienne Randolph, and Alan Morris, "Is Informed Consent Always Necessary for Randomized, Controlled Trials?," *New England Journal of Medicine* 340 (1999): 804–7; Dresser, "Correspondence: Is Informed Consent Always Necessary for Randomized, Controlled Trials?," *New England Journal of Medicine* 341 (1999): 449.
44. Celia Fisher and her colleagues have developed a "co-learning" model that "assumes that experienced or prospective participants have expertise in what they think is important to study, how they have or will react to planned procedures, the subjective risk-benefit balance of the research, and the moral and cultural frameworks informing their perspectives." Celia Fisher, "HIV Prevention Research Ethics: An Introduction to the Special Issue," *Journal of Empirical Research on Human Research Ethics* 9, no. 1 (2014): 1–5, 2.
45. Young, *Inclusion and Democracy*, 119.
46. Ibid., 55. For a review of research on the role of unaffiliated IRB members in research review, see Charles W. Lidz, Lorna J. Simon, Antonia V. Seligowsky et al., "The Participation of Community Members of Medical Institutional Review

Boards," *Journal of Empirical Research on Human Research Ethics* 7, no. 1 (2012): 1–8. In his article contrasting professional with lay ethics review, Veatch predicted that simply including "patient or community representatives will only dilute [professionals'] systematic biases, not eliminate them." Veatch, "Human Experimentation Committees," 37.

47. See Dresser, *When Science Offers Salvation*, 36, 121–23.

2

Personal Knowledge
and Study Participation

■□■

BEFORE THERE WERE ETHICS REVIEW boards, research regulations, the Helsinki Declaration, and the Nuremberg Code, there was self-experimentation. During the nineteenth and much of the twentieth century, many physician-scientists believed self-experimentation was an essential component of ethical research.

One of the best-known examples of self-experimentation involved a team led by the US military physician Walter Reed. In 1900, two of Reed's colleagues allowed themselves to be bitten by mosquitoes to see whether the insects could transmit yellow fever to humans. Both men developed yellow fever, and one died of it.[1] Reed's colleagues were just two of many researchers engaging in self-experimentation.[2] Indeed, the medical school at my university, Washington University in St. Louis, was reportedly nicknamed the "Kamikaze School of Medicine" because of its self-experimentation tradition.[3]

An earlier version of this chapter was published as "Personal Knowledge and Study Participation," *Journal of Medical Ethics* 40 (2014): 471–74.

The Nazi experimentation atrocities and other notorious cases of human subject abuse gave rise to the detailed ethical codes and oversight systems guiding today's research. As the biomedical research enterprise and human subject protection system grew in scope and complexity, self-experimentation faded from the scene. Although accounts of self-experimentation still appear in the literature,[4] the practice plays no significant role in today's research. Neither scientists nor ethicists see self-experimentation as important in contemporary biomedical investigations.

Yet there are good reasons to change this situation. It is time to bring back self-experimentation, albeit in a revised form. Personal experience as a research subject can be eye-opening. Experience as a subject gives one a distinct perspective on the research process, bringing into focus previously overlooked features of human trials. By participating in studies themselves, people in the research community—including those involved in ethical and regulatory oversight—can gain valuable knowledge about the work that they do.

RESEARCH PARTICIPATION—PAST AND PRESENT

In its original guise, self-experimentation was viewed as an "obligation to try a new drug or procedure on oneself."[5] Researchers had both moral and scientific reasons to fulfill this obligation. Self-experimentation was a matter of conscience, a scientific version of the Bible's Golden Rule.[6] Before testing their theories and interventions on other people, scientists thought they ought to expose themselves to experimental hazards. And there was another ethical advantage: self-experimentation involved a subject whose participation was voluntary and informed, someone who was making a truly autonomous choice to accept experimental risks and uncertainties. Writing in 1969, philosopher Hans Jonas praised self-experimentation: "If it is full, autonomous identification of the subject with the [study's] purpose that is required for the dignifying of his serving as a subject—here it is; if strongest motivation—here it is; if fullest understanding—here it is; if freest decision—here it is; if greatest integration with the person's total, chosen pursuit— here it is."[7]

Researchers in the past also thought self-experimentation was educational. It produced good information, for subjects were cooperative, knowledgeable, and alert to the potential effects of an investigational procedure or agent. Scientists found that trying experiments on themselves allowed them "to smooth out the 'bugs' before experimenting on another person," increasing the quality of the investigations that followed.[8] Self-experimentation was a way to earn public trust and support too, for it demonstrated the scientist's genuine commitment to the quest for knowledge.[9]

Because the research environment is now quite different from what it was in earlier times, today we need a modified version of self-experimentation. Self-experimentation is not the best way to evaluate high-risk interventions, for excitement about their ideas can lead self-experimenting researchers to downplay the hazards and burdens, and exaggerate the potential benefits, of such interventions.[10] The modern systems of peer review, regulation, and ethics review are better ways to determine when and how human studies should go forward. But the educational value of self-experimentation endures. Personal experience as a study subject remains a way for researchers to develop a deeper understanding of the ethical dimensions of their work.

THE VALUE OF PERSONAL EXPERIENCE

A growing body of literature describes the new and often surprising professional insights clinicians gain through personal experience as patients.[11] Leading journals feature regular essays by physicians and other health professionals recounting what their experiences with illness have taught them. The increased presence of these narratives is an acknowledgment that personal experience can be a vital component of an individual's professional understanding.[12]

One research field, psychology, has long recognized the educational value of personal participation in studies. Psychology students often participate in research as part of their coursework. Psychology departments adopted this practice partly to produce an adequate subject pool for faculty research. But instructors also see personal research participation as educational for students. And in surveys, many students report that the experience gave them a better understanding of both course content and the research process.[13]

Biomedical fields have yet to adopt this educational method. Similarly, courses on human research ethics fail to recognize the educational value of personal study participation. Certainly some investigators and other research professionals serve as study subjects, but there is no evidence that this practice is common or widespread. One researcher reported: "I teach a lot of classes for research professionals and always ask, 'How many of you have ever participated in a research study?' It's always less than 5 percent of the people in the room and these are people in the industry!"[14] In a book about his experiences as a genetic research subject, Misha Angrist commented, "Scientists who do human subject research spend so much time writing grants, crafting consent forms, collecting samples, experimenting on and analyzing those samples, and then looking for more, that most of us don't have a clue as to how it feels on the other end of the phlebotomist's needle."[15]

Physicians, ethicists, institutional review board (IRB) members, and other research professionals who have been study subjects attest to the educational value of the experience. Physician Jack Coulehan is one of them. He was a junior faculty member when his department head "invited" him to join a vaccine trial. A "sense of duty" and an opportunity to earn a large payment ("easy money") led him to accept the invitation. Later he was told that technical problems made the study samples useless. The investigators stopped their work, and nothing ever came of it. Through personal experience, Coulehan learned that high payment and peer pressure "created a coercive situation." He also learned that research can fall short of expectations, disappointing both the investigators and the subjects who accept pain and other burdens on the assumption that they are making a significant scientific contribution.[16]

Research ethicist Alan Wertheimer learned something similar through personal experience as a study volunteer. After being diagnosed with cancer, Wertheimer agreed to participate in a study of his disease. He consented to join the study because he believed it would generate useful data. (He was eventually excluded, because he failed to meet the study's eligibility criteria.) Two years later, he heard that the study

had been stopped after researchers failed to enroll a sufficient number of subjects. He was startled, for it had never
occurred to him that this could happen—he had volunteered
because he assumed the study would produce worthwhile
information. This experience led Wertheimer to conclude
that researchers should tell prospective subjects when there
is a possibility that low enrollment or other problems could
put a premature end to the study.[17]

Personal experience was quite instructive for Alicia
Pouncey too. Before her father was diagnosed with cancer,
Pouncey had worked in research for many years. Once her
father learned about his diagnosis, he was eager to explore
trial opportunities. After guiding him through a "volumi-
nous consent form," Pouncey realized that what he really
wanted was advice on whether to enroll. He expected the
surgeon describing the trial to tell him what would be best
for him as an individual patient. To her father, there was
no difference between a treating physician and a physician-
investigator conducting a study. As a research professional,
however, Pouncey knew better.[18]

Through personal experience, Pouncey learned how difficult it is for patients to understand research consent forms
and the differences between clinical care and research. She
now believes that trials should have shorter consent forms
and that trial discussions should be led by neutral third
parties, not doctors or others involved in the trial. And she
wishes there were "a way to simulate [risks like] nausea and
vomiting" so that researchers would have a better understanding of what patients go through in trials.[19]

People serving on IRBs have also described what they
learned through becoming study subjects. At a conference
panel discussion involving IRB members, one described his

frustration with the thoroughly uninformative "informed consent" discussion he had experienced. He was tempted to ask the evasive study staff: "Why can't you talk to me as a person? I'm giving you my time—why can't you just talk to me?"[20] Another IRB member who had participated in a vaccine study described how surprised she was when she actually experienced the debilitating flu-like symptoms listed in the risks section of the consent form. Although she had read and understood the information, she hadn't taken it seriously. As she put it, "I was arrogant enough to think it wasn't going to happen to me." She felt terrible, missed a few days of work, and developed a new appreciation of the real-life burdens that trial participation can impose.[21]

WHAT STUDY PARTICIPATION CAN TEACH RESEARCHERS

Personal narratives like these, together with accounts from scientists engaged in self-experimentation, point to several ways in which study participation can educate researchers. By serving as research subjects, investigators and their teams can overcome the professional myopia that makes it hard for researchers to recognize ethical and practical problems with their studies. Participation can give researchers a subject's-eye view of the tests, procedures, and monitoring requirements involved in clinical trials.[22] Participation can help researchers see why individuals might be unwilling to join a trial and why those who do join might later drop out. Researchers with experience as subjects will be better positioned to design and conduct studies that minimize risks and burdens to subjects,[23] which could in turn increase enrollment and retention rates.

Firsthand experience can teach researchers about information disclosure as well. Being on the other side of a study discussion can help researchers recognize deficiencies in their own disclosure methods. Researchers enrolled in trials can see for themselves how incomplete, poorly worded, or overly complex consent forms create difficulties for subjects. Personal experience with such forms can bring home the need to create meaningful and comprehensible documents for their own studies. Researchers who have undergone specific research procedures will also be better equipped to determine what prospective subjects need to know about those procedures.[24]

Though there is no guarantee, it's possible that researchers participating in studies will develop more empathy and concern for their study subjects.[25] In this respect, study participation could foster a "culture of responsibility" in which researchers "understand, internalize, and embrace critical ethical requirements."[26] Moreover, researchers joining studies model the volunteerism they would like to see in others. A commitment by research professionals to serve as subjects would express respect for and solidarity with the thousands of other people who accept the risks and burdens of research participation.

Members of the research community who reject study participation send a less appealing message. It's fair to ask these individuals "whether the lives of patients or research subjects are implicitly devalued against the lives of doctors or scientists."[27] At minimum, researchers unwilling to serve as subjects may appear arrogant and insensitive. That was the case with Chester Southam, a US physician who led the infamous Jewish Chronic Disease Hospital study. In the aftermath of that study, Southam was asked why he failed to expose himself to the same live cancer cells his team had injected into uninformed and debilitated elderly patients. Though Southam insisted the experiment was safe, he revealed his true thoughts when he told an interviewer, "there are relatively few skilled cancer researchers, and it seemed stupid to take even the little risk."[28]

WHAT STUDY PARTICIPATION CAN TEACH OTHER PROFESSIONALS

Participation in studies can be valuable not only to researchers but also to people involved in research oversight. Institutional review board members and staff who have served as subjects say that the experience deepened their understanding of study risks, burdens, and potential benefits. This personal experience strengthened their professional commitment to minimize risks and burdens in the studies they reviewed.[29]

Through serving as subjects, IRB members and staff can develop a better understanding of the information disclosure process as well. Professionals who have had to choose whether to accept study risks and burdens for themselves report finding many problems in consent forms and discussions: Forms were too long and technical, but at the same time omitted important trial information. Research team members were poor communicators and were unable to answer subjects' questions. Through personal experience, professionals became more committed to ensuring that subjects in the studies they reviewed received adequate and accessible information.[30]

Institutional review boards are responsible for promoting informed consent and an acceptable balance of risks and benefits in human research. Members and staff with personal experience as study subjects could reach better decisions on these matters. Overly detailed consent forms might be replaced with more comprehensible documents. There might be fewer misguided study restrictions, and neglected subject vulnerabilities could receive more attention. Complaints about both over- and under-regulation of human research could decrease. Both subjects and researchers could benefit if studies were reviewed by individuals familiar with the realities of research participation.

CONTOURS AND LIMITATIONS

Self-experimentation was once seen as an ethical means to conduct high-risk experiments, but today we have a more scientific and ethically defensible approach to determining when such experiments should go forward. The primary modern rationale for research participation is education.

In light of its modern rationale, contemporary self-experimentation should encompass a wide range of research experiences. Scientists in the past used self-experimentation primarily to evaluate their own research questions, but today's researchers could learn much of what they need to know through joining studies led by others. It's possible that some contemporary investigators would prefer old-style self-experimentation, since it could be particularly instructive. Investigators wishing to participate in their own studies could be permitted to do so if they met the enrollment requirements. Given the potential for undue pressure, however, study coordinators and other junior staff members should not participate in studies led by the investigators employing them.[31]

For similar reasons, institutions and other research organizations should prohibit investigators from directly recruiting anyone working at the same organization. Trial opportunities could be publicized within the organization, but researchers should discuss studies only with employees who initiated contact. That said, everyone on a research team would probably learn the most from participating in studies resembling those that are the focus of their work.

The traditional practice of self-experimentation should be revised in some respects, but self-experimentation should remain a matter of choice. Study participation should be considered a voluntary educational activity. Research professionals should be free to decline study participation and to withdraw from studies if they so choose.[32] Mandating research participation would be ethically objectionable and probably counterproductive as well. Firsthand experience as a study subject should instead be a point of pride, something skilled professionals seek on a regular basis. Members of the research community should regard study participation as a way to demonstrate integrity and achieve excellence in their work.[33]

Given the broad spectrum of clinical research and the variety of study approaches that exist today, it should be possible for everyone to find studies that are personally and medically acceptable. Trials for healthy volunteers would be suitable for many research professionals; some would also qualify for studies addressing specific health conditions. Researchers and other professionals could join studies at their own institutions or at nearby research facilities.[34] Institutions and sponsors could support the effort by collecting and distributing information about local trials seeking subjects. Participation in different types of studies would allow professionals to learn about a variety of research situations.

Of course, personal experience as a study participant cannot give research professionals a full picture of what subjects go through. Professionals must realize that not everyone will experience study participation the same way they do.[35] Members of the research community are unusually well informed about how research works. They also tend to be relatively healthy, well educated, and affluent. As a result, research professionals might not experience the same pressures, risks, burdens, and inconveniences as other subjects. Information learned through personal experience is just one of many ingredients that go into the design and conduct of an ethical human study.

A DUTY TO PARTICIPATE?

We hear a lot these days about the urgent need for patients and healthy volunteers to enroll in clinical trials. Citing this need, certain writers claim that members of the public have a duty to participate in research. Some say this duty is justified by the ethical principles of beneficence and justice,[36] while others contend that knowledge generated through human trials is a public good to which all should contribute.[37] Each argument for a general duty to volunteer hinges on the public health benefits that clinical research generates.

There is no question that members of the public benefit from knowledge gained through clinical research. One can debate whether this benefit is an adequate foundation for a general moral obligation to participate in research.[38] But if benefits from research do create a duty to participate, then the research community has ample reason to volunteer. Besides benefiting from the health advances that research produces, research professionals receive financial and professional benefits from the research enterprise.[39] If the general public has a duty to participate in studies, then the research community has this duty as well.

LEARNING, HUMANIZING, AND LEADING

If more research professionals volunteered to be subjects, there could be material improvement in the conduct and oversight of human research. Empirical studies will be necessary to determine the extent and nature of any benefit produced by this action. (Similar studies are needed to assess the value of the currently accepted methods of teaching researchers and other professionals about human research ethics.) It could be that study participation is as good a way as any to learn about the features of an ethical human study.

Study participation also brings a humanistic element to the "impersonal and mechanistic culture" that characterizes modern human research.[40] Firsthand experience as a study subject offers new insights to individuals whose understanding of research and research ethics comes largely from books, classrooms, and professional interactions. By enrolling in studies, researchers can develop a better understanding of the personal challenges study participants confront. Individuals who have served as research subjects will be more aware of the micro-ethics issues that arise in everyday interactions between researchers and subjects.[41]

Finally, a commitment by research professionals to serve as subjects would fortify the call for greater public participation in trials. Professionals who claim that they are too busy or too indispensable to take on the burdens of study participation cannot complain when ordinary people decline participation for the same reasons. In explaining his support for modern self-experimentation, Lawrence Altman observed, "Scientists like to think of themselves as leaders, and the best way to lead is by example."[42] By serving as study subjects, members of the research community can demonstrate their own willingness to accept personal risks and burdens to improve medical care for future patients.

NOTES

1. Lawrence Altman, *Who Goes First? The Story of Self-Experimentation in Medicine* (Berkeley: University of California Press, 1998), 282; Susan Lederer, "Walter Reed and the Yellow Fever Experiments," in *The Oxford Textbook of Clinical Research Ethics*, ed. Ezekiel Emanuel et al. (New York: Oxford University Press, 2008), 9–17.
2. Susan Lederer, *Subjected to Science: Human Experimentation in the United States Before the Second World War* (Baltimore: Johns Hopkins University Press, 1995).
3. Altman, *Who Goes First?*, 282.
4. Martin Van Der Weyden, "Researchers as Guinea Pigs," *Medical Journal of Australia* 178 (2003): 52–53. Tu Youyou, a 2015 recipient of the Nobel Prize in Medicine, chose to be one of the first humans exposed to an anti-malarial compound she had developed. Jane Perlez, "Answering an Appeal by Mao Led Tu Youyou, a Chinese scientist, to a Nobel Prize," *New York Times*, October 6, 2015. Retrieved November 2, 2015, from http://nyti.ms/1RrQxLr.
5. Lederer, *Subjected to Science*, 18.
6. Altman, *Who Goes First?*, 12.

7. Hans Jonas, "Philosophical Reflections on Experimenting with Human Subjects," *Daedelus* 98, no. 2 (1969): 219–47, 234.

8. Altman, *Who Goes First?*, x.

9. Lederer, *Subjected to Science*, 137–38.

10. John Davis, "Self-Experimentation," *Accountability in Research* 10 (2003): 175–87.

11. Robert Klitzman, *When Doctors Become Patients* (New York: Oxford University Press, 2008).

12. Kieran Sweeney, "Personal Knowledge," *BMJ* 332 (2006): 129–30.

13. Anne Moyer and Nancy Franklin, "Strengthening the Educational Value of Undergraduate Participation in Research as Part of a Psychology Department Pool," *Journal of Empirical Research in Human Research Ethics* 6, no. 1 (2011): 75–82; Jessica Darling et al., "Learning about the Means to the End: What US Introductory Psychology Students Report about Experimental Participation," *Psychology Learning and Teaching* 6, no. 2 (2007): 91–97.

14. See "A Research Professional Learns First-Hand What Matters to Patients," *Global Forum*, August 2010, at 104–105. Retrieved March 6, 2015, from https://www.ciscrp.org/wp-content/uploads/2014/02/Patient_Perspective_Aug2010.pdf. Lawrence Altman believes that self-experimentation occurs "nearly everywhere that research on humans is conducted," though he acknowledges the absence of survey data supporting this belief. Altman, *Who Goes First?*, xii.

15. Misha Angrist, *Here Is a Human Being: At the Dawn of Personal Genomics* (New York: Harper Perennial, 2011), 30.

16. Jack Coulehan, "My Battle against Gonorrhea," *Annals of Internal Medicine* 155 (2011): 198–200.

17. Alan Wertheimer, "Non-completion and Informed Consent," *Journal of Medical Ethics* 40 (2014): 127–30.

18. "A Research Professional," 105.

19. Ibid.

20. Public Responsibility in Medicine & Research, "In Their Own Voices: A Discussion with Research Subjects Who Also Work in the Field of Subject Protections," 2010 Advancing Ethical Research Conference Proceedings. Retrieved March 6, 2015, from https://www.conferencepassport.com/index.asp.

21. Ibid. In a recent essay, bioethicist Dena Davis described what she learned through her participation in a genetic study on Alzheimer's disease risk. Dena Davis, "Ethical Issues in Interpretation of Risk, from the Perspective of a Research Subject," *Narrative Inquiry in Bioethics* 5 (2015): 203–6.

22. S. C. Gandevia, "Self-Experimentation, Ethics and Efficacy," *Monash Bioethics Review* 23, no. 4 (2005): 43–48.

23. Altman, *Who Goes First?*, 303.

24. Altman, *Who Goes First?*, 12, 313; Gandevia, "Self-Experimentation," 45; Kate Mandeville, "My Life as a Guinea Pig," *BMJ* 332 (2006): 735.

25. Ian Kerridge, "Altruism or Reckless Curiosity? A Brief History of Self Experimentation in Medicine," *Internal Medicine Journal* 33 (2003): 203–7.

26. Presidential Commission for the Study of Bioethical Issues, *Moral Science: Protecting Participants in Human Subject Research* (December 2011), 72. Retrieved March 6, 2015, from http://www.bioethics.gov/cms/node/558.

27. Kerridge, "Altruism or Reckless Curiosity?," 206.

28. Altman, *Who Goes First?*, 297.

29. Public Responsibility in Medicine & Research, "In Their Own Voices."

30. Ibid.

31. Ibid.; Allen Cheng, "'Self-Experimentation' in Vulnerable Populations," *Medical Journal of Australia* 178 (2003): 471.

32. See Karen Schwenzer, "Protecting Vulnerable Subjects in Clinical Research: Children, Pregnant Women, Prisoners, and Employees," *Respiratory Care* 53 (2008): 1342–49.

33. Ibid.

34. Public Responsibility in Medicine & Research, "In Their Own Voices."

35. Sarah Greene, Kathleen Mazor, and Thomas Gallagher, "Participating in Biomedical Research," *JAMA* 302 (2009): 2200; Carisa Cunningham, "Scientists Discuss Experiments on Self," *Harvard Gazette*, April 29, 2004. Retrieved March 5, 2015, from http://news.harvard.edu/gazette/2004/04.29/11-selfexperiment.html. A 1939 essay written by a self-experimenting scientist is proof that self-experimentation does not always make scientists sensitive to subjects or to

ethical considerations in research. See W. Oslter Abbott, "The Problem of the Professional Guinea Pig," *Transactions of the American Clinical and Climatological Association* 68 (1957): 1–9.

36. John Harris, "Scientific Research Is a Moral Duty," *Journal of Medical Ethics* 31 (2005): 242–48.

37. G. Owen Schaefer, Ezekiel Emanuel, and Alan Wertheimer, "The Obligation to Participate in Biomedical Research," *JAMA* 302 (2009): 67–72.

38. Stuart Rennie, "Viewing Research Participation as a Moral Obligation: In Whose Interests?," *Hastings Center Report* 41, no. 2 (2011): 40–47.

39. Greene, Mazor, and Gallagher et al., "Participating in Biomedical Research," 2200.

40. Van Der Weyden, "Researchers as Guinea Pigs," 53.

41. Debra Debruin, Joan Liaschenko, and Anastasia Fisher, "How Clinical Trials Really Work: Rethinking Research Ethics," *Kennedy Institute of Ethics Journal* 21 (2011): 121–39.

42. Altman, *Who Goes First?*, 315.

3

The Everyday Ethics
of Human Research

■□■

IN THEIR 2013 BOOK *What Patients Teach: The Everyday Ethics of Health Care*, Larry Churchill, Joseph Fanning, and David Schenk describe how patients experience medical care. Drawing on in-depth conversations with patients, Churchill and his colleagues develop a patient-centered medical ethics. They identify both "clinician traits that heal,"[1] such as attentiveness, honesty, and empathy, and clinican behavior that harms, such as poor communication and treating patients as objects or numbers rather than as valued individuals.

From the patient's point of view, ethical care is important not just in dramatic life-and-death situations but also in everyday medical encounters. *What Patients Teach* contends that medical ethics has neglected the ethics of routine care. Churchill and his coauthors argue that the conventional preoccupation with ethical principles "leads us away from the heart of the routine moral activity between clinicians and patients." In emphasizing abstract ethical principles,

An earlier version of this chapter was published as "What Subjects Teach: The Everyday Ethics of Human Research," *Wake Forest Law Review* 50 (2015): 301–41.

the authors say, conventional medical ethics "runs the risk of becoming irrelevant."[2]

Besides neglecting the ethics of routine medical care, traditional medical ethics relies too heavily on what professionals, rather than patients, see as ethical care. Churchill and his coauthors criticize the "narcissism" of medical ethics codes. Such codes "originate in the perceptions of the professionals themselves, with little or no influence from patients' understanding of what is at stake in the therapeutic encounter."[3] Similarly, lists of patients' ethical responsibilities tend to reflect medical professionals' moral judgments, excluding patients' own views on the matter.

Many of the points Churchill and his colleagues make about medical ethics apply equally to research ethics. A research ethics that neglects subjects' perspectives has flaws resembling those of the principle-based medical ethics criticized in *What Patients Teach*. Conventional research ethics largely overlooks the everyday encounters that determine how subjects experience their participation. Existing codes and principles of research ethics also reflect professional narcissism. For the most part, research ethics has developed without serious attention to the views of people who know what it is like to be a research subject.

This chapter examines subjects' perspectives on study participation. It describes how healthy volunteers and patients perceive the potential benefits and harms of participation and how they decide whether or not to enroll in trials. It also describes what parents and surrogates experience when deciding whether to enroll children and cognitively disabled adults in studies.

Whenever possible, I draw on reports of open-ended interviews and other qualitative investigations that allow subjects to bring up the concerns and experiences they consider relevant and important. Such investigations offer different insights from what one finds in questionnaires and surveys, which are shaped by the interests and awareness of the research teams creating them. Studies using closed-ended questions can keep people from supplying full accounts of their research experiences. As a result, study findings "may reflect the views and interests of the researchers," as opposed to those of the subjects themselves.[4] My objectives are to highlight subjects' voices, describe "how it actually feels to be the subject of clinical research,"[5] and determine how subjects "make sense of the total experience of trial participation, from recruitment to follow-up."[6]

The available information on subject perspectives is less robust than one would like. For example, the literature contains much less information about people who decline study participation than about those who consent to it. There is also a dearth of information about the views of patients whose conditions deteriorate during and after study participation. The reasons for this scarcity are unclear, but it may stem from a reluctance to bother patients dealing with worsening health problems. (One team reported that an ethics committee refused to allow interviews with cancer patients whose condition failed to improve despite receiving treatment in a trial.[7]) Data about trial decliners and trial participants with bad outcomes would be quite valuable in ethical and policy deliberations about human research. Studies of these groups are needed to "more fully represent perceptions and understandings of trial participants."[8]

There are two general categories of human research: studies involving healthy or "normal" volunteers, and studies involving people with medical conditions, who are often referred to as patient-subjects. Below I describe how healthy volunteers and patient-subjects evaluate research benefits and burdens in making research decisions.

SUBJECTS' PERSPECTIVES: HEALTHY VOLUNTEERS

Research Benefits

Most healthy volunteers see monetary compensation as the major benefit of research participation. In interviews and questionnaires, many volunteers say that payment is the main reason they become research subjects.[9]

Compensation is most important to people who participate in studies on a regular basis.[10] For many of these repeat volunteers, study participation is an important income source. These "professional guinea pigs" see themselves as motivated by the same considerations as the researchers who make a living from their study involvement.[11] Volunteers in this group also tend to think that study payment should be higher than it is, dismissing ethicists' concern that high payments make study participation too tempting to people who need money.[12]

Although many healthy volunteers see compensation as the major benefit of study participation, they name other benefits too. Some say they want to contribute to scientific knowledge and healthcare improvements.[13] Some are attracted by the health examinations and tests that subjects receive in many studies.[14] Repeat volunteers say that study participation seems safer and more interesting than other employment options.[15] Additional motivating factors include curiosity, a desire to meet people or take a break from the routine,[16] and interest in learning "what's new in the medical field."[17]

Volunteers want to participate in studies that produce useful information and have real benefit to others.[18] Many see themselves as essential contributors to research. Because they believe they have a stake in the studies they join, they believe they should have an opportunity to learn about study results.[19] Many also think that compensation is recognition of their essential role. For them, rather than being exploitative, "money in some respects serve[s] to equalize an otherwise highly imbalanced exchange."[20]

Experienced volunteers look for studies conducted by people they can trust, people who treat them with respect and understanding. They value courteous and skilled research staff members who appreciate what subjects do and pay attention to their well-being.[21] For example, one volunteer expressed delight when a nurse praised her commitment to study requirements.[22] Another volunteer advised researchers: "Be approachable. Don't be judgmental. Hear what we have to say. Honestly listen to it."[23]

Volunteers participating in studies that require them to live in research facilities for long periods value comfortable quarters, decent food, and entertaining pastimes. For example, one volunteer commended a study staff that "bent over backward to get us anything we wanted, from books and hard-to-find movies to hoagie sandwiches from my favorite deli for Superbowl Sunday and a bowl of garlic when I felt a cold coming on."[24] Although matters like these may seem trivial, subjects see them as expressions of researchers' respect and concern for their welfare.[25]

Research Harms

Certain study features attract healthy individuals to research participation, but other features are not so appealing. Studies expose participants to physical and psychological risks. Conventional approaches to research ethics and regulation take many of these hazards into account, but experienced volunteers point to burdens that others in the research enterprise rarely acknowledge.[26]

Some volunteers have written vivid accounts that highlight overlooked study burdens. In one such account, a science journalist described her participation in a week-long study of the brain's response to temporary blindness. Contrary to researchers' assurances, study procedures were far from "quick and easy." One of her MRI scans was delayed by a broken machine, requiring her to "lie still for what seem[ed] like hours." Adjusting to sightlessness was difficult, too—she cut her lip while trying to walk and "saw" unsettling images while wearing the blindfold the study required. Other incidents left her anxious, alarmed, and feeling vulnerable, so that after a few days she was "so ready for this to end." Once the blindfold was removed, it took time for her vision to return; when it did, she started "to cry with relief."[27]

As this personal account shows, what may on paper appear as undemanding study requirements can actually be quite burdensome to participants. Another healthy volunteer made this point about the yearly memory tests that were part of an Alzheimer's disease study. Such tests are usually considered low-burden research procedures. But this volunteer found the tests unexpectedly stressful, because he kept wondering whether his performance was satisfactory. This made him realize that the tests could be even more upsetting to someone with memory problems.[28] A journalist wrote that the healthy volunteer he interviewed regarded a schixophrenia study's eighteen hours of neuropsychological testing as "anything but 'noninvasive.' Instead it was invasive in a way that was more insidious than if someone had stuck a tube down [the volunteer's] throat."[29]

Volunteers also point to personal hardships imposed by outwardly insignificant study demands. They call attention to the "nontrivial" time required to participate in studies, as well as the need to arrange child care and transportation.[30] Studies may also involve embarrassing examinations and procedures, along with restrictions on ordinary activities.[31] Study schedule changes can be a major inconvenience for volunteers.[32] And the side effects of study drugs can leave subjects unable to work, leading to income loss.[33]

Repeat volunteers complain about the tedium of studies requiring overnight stays. One participant in a two-week study wrote that the study unit "had this desperate, *Flowers in the Attic* feeling." She and the other volunteers would "look out the window and watch people do their normal, everyday errands."[34] Another described his state of mind as follows: "I feel that I am a worker but it is not work, it's like a security guard that does not produce something, just watches stuff. A security guard just gets paid to be bored, it's about how much you can deal with being bored, that's the real hard part of it, the time and discomfort of being there."[35]

The study environment has a significant impact on subjects' well-being.[36] Just as courteous treatment and pleasant surroundings improve things for study volunteers, rudeness and unpleasant surroundings make things worse. Volunteers complain about conditions like cold waiting rooms and inedible food. Rude behavior by people conducting research is a common theme in volunteer complaints. In one focus group, women with a history of illegal drug use criticized researchers for "acting superior" and "talking down and being condescending."[37] Other volunteers report that researchers treated them as data sources rather than as people. As one volunteer put it, "they don't care about what you are thinking and they don't want to be talked about, they just want your body to do something and react to the drug so they can watch it."[38]

Disorganized and inattentive research staff add burdens beyond those imposed by study requirements. One volunteer wrote of her extreme anxiety, racing thoughts, and sleeplessness while taking a study drug. She tried to reach someone on the research team, but had to leave several messages and wait a week for a return call. Later a staff member apologized, explaining that she had been on vacation and her substitute had turned off the pager. At that point, the volunteer wrote, "I knew exactly what was going on—nobody cared."[39] Eventually she received a call from a study doctor, who said that symptoms like hers "sometimes" diminished over time. The doctor ended the call without offering any follow-up care.

How Healthy Volunteers Decide

When deciding whether to enroll in studies, healthy volunteers weigh the potential benefits and harms of participation. Risk is the main reason volunteers turn down studies.[40] Yet it's not clear that all volunteers appreciate the risks they are facing. A journalist wrote that the student volunteers she interviewed didn't worry about adverse events: "They're young, healthy, and suffering from a shared condition. They believe they're invulnerable."[41] Few volunteers interviewed after the unexpected death of a healthy subject worried about their safety. Most thought, without any supporting evidence, that the subject must have contributed to what happened by failing to ask enough questions or to follow study requirements.[42]

Some volunteers admit that the prospect of compensation trumps their reservations about study risks. One volunteer explained, "You become addicted to the easy money, you don't want to do anything else."[43] Another volunteer said, "If there were a study where they cut off your leg and sewed it back on and you got twenty thousand dollars, people would be fighting to get into that study."[44]

According to existing ethics guidelines, payment to volunteers should reflect the time and inconvenience a study involves, rather than the level of risk.[45] But many subjects think higher risk justifies higher payment.[46] For example, women participating in an imaging study agreed that study time and inconvenience should determine payment amounts. But most women thought payment should reflect the unknown risks of research interventions too. One woman said: "If the product is experimental, the reimbursement should be more. . . . Because you're basically a guinea pig, so you're putting yourself at risk for something."[47] When a different group of experienced subjects was asked about compensation, 65 percent said the level of risk should affect the amount of payment.[48]

Interviews and studies reveal that volunteers don't always see research the way researchers and other nonparticipants do. Although research participation is usually portrayed as an altruistic activity, most volunteers believe they are entitled to compensation. Indeed, most are unwilling to participate without compensation. And like the patients in *What Patients Teach*, research volunteers give close attention to both kindnesses and slights that occur in routine interactions with professionals conducting studies. They describe study burdens that researchers and other outsiders don't always recognize. Some admit that their desire for payment leads them to disregard study risks. On these and other matters, volunteers have distinct perspectives on the ethics of human research.

SUBJECTS' PERSPECTIVES: PATIENT-SUBJECTS

Research Benefits

Potential health benefits are the main reason patients participate in research. In a questionnaire study, 42 percent of cancer trial participants said that potential medical benefit was their single most important reason for enrolling, with no other reason coming close.[49] A survey of and interviews with cancer trial participants found that nearly all of them were motivated by hope for direct medical benefit.[50] A researcher reported that more than half the cancer trial participants she interviewed "described the offer of the trial as being 'the light at the end of the tunnel,' because of the hope it offered. This included hoping that the trial treatment would be a miracle cure, that it would be better than current treatment, that they might achieve relief of symptoms, and that they would live longer."[51] Interviews with patients suffering from pulmonary hypertension produced similar findings. More than half the patients hoped trial enrollment would result in personal health benefit.[52] In another set of interviews, patients who had participated in a variety of studies cited hope for personal benefit, such as "access to what would become the new gold standard or the miracle drug," as their reason for enrolling.[53]

Patients join studies to obtain other personal benefits. Some are attracted by the prospect of "increased physical surveillance, including additional clinic visits," that goes along with trial participation; they believe this surveillance can supply potentially useful information about their health.[54] Certain studies offer patient-subjects financial compensation, and some patients say they are more likely to enroll in such studies.[55] Almost all patient-subjects see the opportunity to learn about study results as an important benefit of participation.[56]

Patients also participate in research for altruistic reasons. For many, participation is a way to help others coping with disease. But as noted above, potential health benefits, not altruism, are the main reason most patients enroll in trials. An assessment of cancer trial participants found that "although approximately half of respondents identified altruism as a very important motivation, less than 1 in 7 reported that altruism was their primary reason for joining the trial."[57] Strikingly, patients in early-phase trials that rarely provide personal medical benefit were least likely to be motivated by altruism.[58]

Patients have a few other reasons for enrolling in studies. Some report that the opportunity to enroll "made them feel special, privileged, pleased, lucky and honoured, because, as they described it, 'not everyone gets the chance to take part in something like this.'"[59] Participants in HIV trials saw "trials as an opportunity to empower themselves in their fight against the disease, a way to take control of their bodies and their lives."[60] Some patients also enroll because they want to help doctors who cared for them.[61]

Research Harms

Patients don't have a completely positive view of study participation. Those hoping for medical benefit are deterred from enrolling by research requirements that seem to reduce this possibility. Randomization requirements can be especially disturbing to patients. Most experts see randomization as an ethically acceptable method of assigning subjects to a study intervention as long as all of the study interventions are in clinical equipoise. Clinical equipoise exists when experts are uncertain about which intervention is best for patients with a particular condition. When clinical equipoise exists, patients randomly assigned to any study intervention have an equal chance of receiving the intervention that will be best for them.[62]

But many patients find it difficult to accept the medical uncertainty underlying randomization and clinical equipoise. They are troubled to learn that doctors don't know which drug or other treatment would be best for them. Such patients often develop a belief that one of the study interventions is better than the others.[63] Usually patients prefer a new intervention over existing ones, because they assume the new one must be better.[64]

Empirical studies reveal how patients think about randomization. A team conducting interviews with men asked to participate in a trial evaluating treatments for benign prostatic disease found that most of the men had a hard time accepting randomization. For those men, understanding the trial's design features, including randomization, "did not ... mean that such concepts made sense or were believable." To make sense of the trial, men used different strategies. "Some became distrustful, because of assumptions about the existence of rationing, others put their trust in their clinicians and their beliefs about fate and destiny, while others just keep struggling with the perceived inconsistencies." One man "wanted the doctors to tell him what treatment would be most suitable for him and perceived the trial to be a 'trick.'" Several of the men who refused to participate did so because they wanted to receive a specific form of treatment.[65]

Interviews with potential cancer trial participants yielded similar findings. Almost all patients were unsettled by the prospect of being randomly assigned to a treatment. Some patients also saw randomization as unethical. One patient explained her reaction this way: "When do we draw lots? We do that when we have a lottery or we gamble, I mean—when we take a risk, and that's not compatible with what doctors should stand for. They should stand for trustworthiness, safety, and 'we take over' and 'we are able' .... [T]he trusting relationship between doctor and patient suffers."[66] Another one of the patients said, "it's all wrong to start with a drawing of lots, because you really want to be in safe surroundings and be told that the treatment you're going to have will help you. And you don't feel that with a drawing of lots."[67]

Randomized trials that include a placebo-control group are the hardest for patients to accept. Placebo-control groups are generally seen as ethically acceptable in certain circumstances, such as when there is no proven treatment for the subjects' condition.[68] But patients often refuse to participate in placebo-controlled trials. Some who do agree to participate drop out if they think they are in the placebo group. (For more discussion of this phenomenon, see chapter 4.) These patients find it difficult to accept that assignment to a placebo group might actually turn out to be best for them.[69]

Good illustrations of this thinking come from an interview study involving patients with Parkinson's disease. Surgical interventions for this condition are typically tested against a placebo, in this case a "sham" surgical procedure. Some of the patients who were interviewed questioned the necessity of including a placebo group, asking whether there were alternative ways to evaluate the study intervention. For example, one said, "If it was a good operation and the results gave big improvements, I don't see why you'd need a placebo group in that case." Another who accepted the scientific need for the placebo felt its use was dehumanizing: "you take on the semblance of something in a Petri dish, rather than a person."[70] Many saw the use of a placebo as unfair because it would expose subjects to a surgical procedure with no possibility of direct benefit.

Besides distress and even anger at research requirements for randomization and control groups, patients worry about the risks involved in exposure to a relatively untested intervention.[71] Fear can be especially strong among patients with serious illnesses. Such feelings were evident in one group's interviews with cancer patients. Some patients declined trial participation because they were "scared of the unknown." According to the researchers, the "graver the patients evaluated their situation the more they wanted to do the right thing and consequently also the more negatively they assessed any factor imposing risk or uncertainty."[72]

At times, patients coping with a serious diagnosis find that enrolling in a trial "is just too much to think about."[73] People with generally positive attitudes toward research can become more cautious and skeptical when facing a personal research decision. This happened to me when I was a cancer patient invited to join a trial. My feelings resembled those of another patient who declined participation in a different trial: "It was a shocking experience to realise that now it was personal and I couldn't participate. I was shocked that I couldn't contribute in helping others. . . . I would very much have liked to do that, but I wasn't capable of it."[74]

Some patients are also repelled by what they perceive as the research team's impersonal manner. One health professional with serious cancer had this reaction. She initially thought she would enroll in a trial, but after being screened for eligibility, she changed her mind. In contrast to her own doctor's "compassion and empathy," the "competent and professional" study investigators seemed "oddly disconnected from the fact that she was a woman told she might be facing a death sentence."[75] Because she "felt experimented on," rather than "cared for," she decided against trial participation.

The practical aspects of trial participation can present problems for patients too. Like healthy volunteers, patient-subjects are expected to arrange their lives around study requirements. But patients can be particularly ill-equipped to deal with study demands. As one writer put it, "often clinical trials are aptly named: they are trials—difficult and exhausting, at a time when a patient's physical and emotional capacities are already stretched thin."[76] In interviews, 65 percent of patients with pulmonary hypertension said that time demands, travel requirements, and other inconveniences could deter them from participating in studies.[77] People with mental health disorders cited travel distance, time away from work, and lack of flexible schedules as reasons for declining participation.[78] Because research participation can generate extra costs for patients, some don't enroll because they can't afford the added expense.[79]

Patients who do enroll in trials may change their minds after dealing with study demands such as travel, visits, tests, and hospital stays. In one study, common reasons for dropping out early were time constraints and disorganization among the study staff.[80] Some subjects in poor health told interviewers that completing trial surveys was tiring and that their survey responses were unwelcome evidence of their continuing decline. At times, "the cumulative effects of relatively trivial burdens led to dissatisfaction and even alienation, particularly for debilitated individuals."[81] In interviews, some experienced subjects said they wouldn't participate in any more studies because they were dissatisfied with aspects of previous trials. For example, one former subject said, "I would have liked to have a better understanding of how I was going to feel."[82]

Cancer trial participants can become particularly disillusioned. One research team reported that patients in cancer trials "are disappointed not to learn more about their disease through their involvement in research and they find that trial participation takes more time and effort than they thought it would."[83] A qualitative study of cancer trial participants found that all had "an increasing sense of being burdened" as the trial proceeded. Patients often wondered "why they were putting themselves through the trial in the first place, and whether it was all worthwhile." Many became disheartened and antagonistic, saying things like "I shouldn't feel like this because the results have been so good for me—you know the [tumor] shrinkage has been great. I should be feeling more encouraged than I am. I don't know. It's got to be a real drag coming here." Another subject complained: "We can't plan anything. I feel as though I'm not in control of my life at all. All I see is hospitals, white coats and nurses."[84] Most of the patients decided to stay in the trial despite their negative feelings, but researchers eventually removed 70 percent of them because they suffered serious side effects or their cancer progressed. When this happened, patients were upset and disappointed.

There is also evidence that patient-subjects care about the commercial aspects of research. In interviews, experienced subjects criticized trials conducted primarily to generate profits, such as trials of "me-too" drugs or those aimed at extending a drug's patent protection. One subject put it this way: "I assume it is on the up and up and not so that [the pharmaceutical company] can make a million dollars marketing the drug. [I]f I am in the guinea pig group, I want to make sure . . . I am not sacrificing my body for someone's bottom line."[85]

The experienced subjects in that interview study also wanted to know more about the compensation investigators receive for conducting research. A brief mention that researchers are compensated wasn't enough for at least some subjects—they wanted to know how much the researchers would earn. One subject said: "[W]hen there is something like that statement in the consent form—'the researcher is getting compensated'—I would think it was like $10—not anything big. It wouldn't occur to me. The way it is written it's like they want you to gloss over it."[86] Researchers ought to disclose these details, another subject said, as "a matter of respect" for the individuals taking part in a study.[87]

These experienced subjects also criticized researchers who failed to inform them of study results. As the interview team reported, many subjects "were disappointed that they had not been re-contacted and informed about study results as was promised or anticipated when enrolling." This research omission, subjects said, reduced their interest in participating in future studies.[88] Similarly, a large survey of experienced subjects found that 72 percent considered information on research results a "very important" factor in their willingness to join future studies.[89]

How Patient-Subjects Decide

Like healthy volunteers, patients making research decisions evaluate the potential benefits and harms of participation. But patients have a certain mindset that can shape their understanding of trial information. As one interview team reported, "data suggest that participants' beliefs and expectations about healthcare may make it difficult for them to absorb key information when trying to make informed decisions about participating in research."[90]

Many patients exhibit what ethicists call the "therapeutic misconception" about research. These patients fail to understand that research participation is different from receiving ordinary medical care.[91] Some patients believe that research is governed by concern for their individual best interests, when it is in fact governed by the need to gather accurate and useful data to guide the care of future patients.[92] In research, decisions about subjects' treatment will be based on scientific needs, rather than on what physicians think would be best for them as individuals. Patients' failure to understand the nature and goals of research can lead them to overestimate the chance that they will obtain personal medical benefit from enrolling in a trial.[93]

Besides a general misunderstanding of research requirements, patients may misunderstand how research rules and goals will apply specifically to them. Some patient-subjects appear to understand subjects' overall chance of medical benefit in a particular trial, but mistakenly believe that certain factors give them a higher-than-average chance of receiving such a benefit.[94] Ethicists refer to this bias as "unrealistic optimism."[95]

A team interviewing parents considering whether to enroll their children in a phase 1 cancer trial described an example of this thinking. A mother thought that her son had a relatively high chance of benefit because he had previously been helped by a drug similar to the one the trial was testing. But the mother failed to recognize that other children in the trial might also have been helped by drugs resembling the study drug. Thus her reason for believing her son was exceptional lacked a firm basis in reality.[96]

Unrealistic optimism desn't fully account for subjects' hope for medical benefit, however. Even patients with a realistic view of their trial prospects may maintain high hopes for medical improvement. In one interview study, cancer trial participants who overestimated their chance of personal benefit said they were not making a factual statement but were "expressing their hope or a positive attitude."[97] Another group of cancer trial participants said that their high expectations were based on their belief that optimism can have positive health effects, on their desire to keep fighting their disease, or on their faith in religion, science, or doctors. Some participants also explained that they were trying to behave in ways that would please "the medical community, their families, and even their faith networks."[98]

Besides overestimating the chance of direct medical benefit, patients may underestimate study risks. Such underestimates are often related to unrealistic optimism: subjects believe that their personal risk is lower than the risk faced by other study subjects. Risk underestimates can also reflect a participant's failure to understand or attend to trial information. One group found that only 3 percent of trial subjects recognized that research involved special burdens, such as extra biopsies and other procedures. This finding "supports the concern that participants either do not understand or do not focus on the key differences between individual care and research."[99]

In other interviews, some experienced patient-subjects characterized participation as a way to "give back with no real risk at all." Some of these subjects didn't take risk information seriously, instead believing that risk disclosure was "a formality—like what you sign before surgery, the form saying you might die. It was just like the legal language thing on the consent forms." Some also said that the government would not permit, and doctors would not recommend, any study that presented serious risks to participants.[100]

As these remarks suggest, trust in clinicians and the medical system plays a big role in patients' willingness to participate in research. In interviews, experienced subjects said they assumed that doctors would not suggest or recommend trial participation if it were not the best option for them. Some assumed that trials conducted in hospitals or other medical facilities must be beneficial for patients.[101] Some said it would be difficult to say no if a doctor they trusted asked them to consider study participation.[102]

Given how much many patients trust doctors, it's not surprising that such patients want doctors to tell them what choice to make. For example, nearly 80 percent of the cancer trial participants in one qualitative study said they wanted a doctor's recommendation on whether to enroll.[103] In interviews, many women considering cancer trial participation said that because their knowledge was inadequate, they "would have preferred the doctor to make that choice for them."[104] One woman said: "I was really surprised that they put me in that situation with such a serious disease, [wanting] me to make choices about my own disease. It had an incredible effect on me, I felt bad about it, and I couldn't get the doctor to just give me . . . advice."[105]

For many patients, clinical trial participation is a confusing and unnerving variation on the medical care they are familiar with. The shift from ordinary clinical care to the different and usually foreign territory of research takes people by surprise. Making research decisions in the context of serious illness is also emotionally demanding. The pressures and distractions of serious illness make it difficult for people to learn what they need to know. It can be hard for patients to understand the differences between research and medical care, and patients who do understand the differences want to believe that their prospects are better than those of other trial subjects. Patients' experiences expose research burdens that are easy for outsiders to overlook, and they show how serious illness can shape subjects' attitudes and responses to research.

Deciding for Others

Some people don't make their own research choices. Parents decide whether their children participate in studies. Surrogate decision makers, typically family members, decide for adults with mentally disabling conditions like dementia. Besides facing many of the same problems that adult research subjects face, parents and surrogates confront distinct challenges. Parents and surrogates operate with a heavy sense of responsibility for their loved ones. They blame themselves for any bad consequences that follow their decisions. Parents and surrogates must also factor in the views of the prospective subjects they are responsible for.

Parents and Children

Parents are legally authorized to make research decisions for their children. This can be a heavy burden, especially for parents whose children are seriously ill. Parents considering research want to make the best possible choices for their children, but fear they won't succeed. Mothers of children enrolled in a bone marrow transplantation study said they "dreaded the possibility that they might have to live with the knowledge that they had made the 'wrong' decision and this was intensified when things did not go well for the child."[106] Another group of parents said it would be much harder to make research decisions for their children than to make those decisions for themselves.[107]

Parents can also be extremely cautious about exposing their children to research risks. In a survey of new parents, one-third said they would be more reluctant to accept certain research risks for their children than to accept those risks for themselves.[108] Parents also assess risks differently than health professionals do. As two scholars observed, "To the clinician research can be considered low risk when it involves no greater risk than conventional treatment. To the parent everything is high risk because they have a sick child."[109]

Potential medical benefit is the overwhelming reason parents agree to a child's research participation. In a questionnaire study, 100 percent of parents of sick children said direct benefit to the child would be the main reason to enroll the child in research.[110] Parents often list altruism as one of their motivations for agreeing to trials, but many do so only after being prompted to consider whether altruism played a role.[111] In discussing research participation for his son with cancer, one father openly admitted his priority: although he knew that researchers focus on helping patients as a group, when parents like him face a research choice, "it's all about the one."[112]

Like adult patients facing research decisions, parents are often troubled by randomization. Parents seeking the best treatment for their children are alarmed to discover that in clinical trials, chance determines a child's treatment. Many parents do not understand randomization; in one study this was true of 50 percent of parents deciding about their children's participation in cancer trials.[113] Other parents understand that randomization is a way of assigning subjects to different interventions, but fail to understand or accept its scientific rationale. In interviews, some parents said that randomization was a way to allow parents and doctors to avoid the burden of choosing among treatments. Some said it was a way to ration interventions that could not be provided to all children. And some concluded that randomization allowed their child to receive the best intervention.[114]

Many parents are also anxious and distracted when making research decisions. The mother of a child with a brain tumor described how she and her husband felt during a study discussion: "We were an emotional wreck. . . . Both of us were nodding our heads and didn't hear a damn word [the doctors] said." It was almost impossible to concentrate on the information, she said, because she and her husband were grieving the loss of their healthy son as they made their decisions.[115] Other parents considering study participation for seriously ill children report similar distress—distress that can keep them from actively participating in study discussions.[116] In interviews conducted after parents had met with researchers, parents asked many questions and raised many concerns they had not voiced in the earlier study discussion.[117]

Parents struggle to reconcile their protective responsibilities with their dependence on clinicans. One mother of a child with hemophilia described her reaction to being approached about enrolling her son in a trial. She worried that declining trial participation would damage her relationships with the clinicians who cared for her son: "You've become really reliant on these people, and they are asking you to participate in this study. . . . The last thing you want to do is tick these people off."[118]

Many parents seek clinicians' advice on enrollment, yet few want to transfer their decision-making authority to clinicians. For example, one group of parents who agreed to their children's trial participation said that even though the choice was difficult, "they felt it was theirs to make."[119] In several surveys, almost all parents said they did not want clinicians to take responsibility for this choice.[120]

Another factor is the child's opinion on research participation. Guidelines and regulations promote children's involvement in the choice, giving children the power to veto participation in certain circumstances. Studies show that children themselves want to be involved,[121] and many parents agree with this. For example, a mother considering research for her six-year-old said that even children this young should have an opportunity to ask questions about research options. "They might not have any," she said, "but they're so happy to be asked."[122]

At the same time, children and parents may have different opinions on when participation is appropriate. For example, when a group of parents and children were asked about hypothetical research participation, almost twice as many children as parents expressed a willingness to enroll in higher-risk trials.[123] When there is disagreement about participation, parents may urge their children to reconsider or may overrule the children altogether.

Parents are most likely to question or dismiss a child's reluctance to participate when a trial seems to offer potential medical benefit. For example, parents of children with chronic medical conditions like diabetes said they would not hesitate to persuade their children to join studies offering potential medical benefit.[124] In interviews, nearly half of a group of children in cancer trials said they had played no part or very little part in the enrollment decision. Thirty-eight percent of the children who were interviewed said they did not feel free to object to participation, usually because they felt pressure from their parents, doctors, or both.[125]

Surrogates and Cognitively Impaired Adults

Research decisions for adults with cognitive impairments present their own distinct challenges. Surrogates' legal authority to decide for cognitively impaired adults is not clearly established in some jurisdictions. Surrogate decision-making is also complex, for in most cases the potential research subject was once a fully functioning adult with specific values and preferences. It's not always clear how those values and preferences should influence research choices. Laws and ethical guidelines often instruct surrogates to give first priority to the incapable adult's former views, but empirical evidence suggests that most surrogates take a different approach.

Most studies of surrogate decision-making in research focus on dementia research. As in other research contexts, the most common reason for enrolling people with dementia is to help the patient. In one set of interviews, 80 percent of surrogates cited this reason; 53 percent cited altruistic reasons.[126] Surrogates also report having the same sense of heightened responsibility that parents do. In interviews, for example, some surrogates said they were reluctant to consent to research because they "would not want to feel regret if they did make the choice and a bad outcome occurred to the patient."[127] Another surrogate observed, "it's very different when you're thinking about it for somebody else than for yourself."[128]

Mainstream legal and ethical standards instruct surrogates to make the choice an incapable patient would make if he or she were capable of choosing (a standard known as "substituted judgment"). But studies show that surrogates are equally or more focused on protecting the patient's current well-being (a standard known as "best interests"). For example, one team asked surrogates for Alzheimer's disease patients how they would decide whether to enroll the patients in clinical trials. The majority of surrogates said that their primary consideration would be the patient's best interests, although they would also consider what the patient would choose.[129] A different research team found similar results when examining decision-making by the "study partners" of research participants with mild-to-moderate Alzheimer's. Fifty-nine percent of the study partners said that research decisions should maximize the patient's well-being. Just 24 percent said decisions should be based on what the patient would want if he or she were competent. The remaining 17 percent saw no difference in the two approaches, because they assumed patients would want what was best for them now.[130]

Many surrogates say that they rely heavily on the patient's current preferences, as opposed to past preferences, to guide research decision-making. One team reported, "Unexpectedly, we found that honoring their relatives' *current* wishes was explicitly emphasized by many of the [surrogates] interviewed, who often distinguished these from premorbid preferences."[131] Moreover, a collaborative process of choosing often occurs even when patients' abilities are impaired. For example, a group of investigators examining research decision-making for people with Alzheimer's found that incapable patients were just as likely to be involved in research decisions as were patients who were still mentally able to choose for themselves.[132]

In interviews, some surrogates also distinguished the patient's former self from his or her present self, voicing greatest allegiance to the present self. For example, one surrogate said:

> The situation is that there was a person there that kind of went away and can't judge for themselves anymore, so you could either judge from their past self, before they had Alzheimer's, or you could judge from their present selves, or you could judge from their future selves. And, mostly, I kind of center around their present self. And so I think that whatever is making that person happy right now is what I should be centering my decisions on.[133]

Another surrogate said of her mother with Alzheimer's, "If she wasn't already compromised, she might think like, 'Oh, this is, you know, I would like to help.' But she just doesn't have that tolerance anymore."[134] Even the surrogates who assigned priority to a patient's past preferences said their research decisions would take into account any risks, discomfort, or distress that would affect patients in their current state. Others "explicitly described the need to weigh numerous factors concurrently—including their relative's preferences and personality before becoming ill, possible benefits to society, possible discomfort to their loved one, and current quality of life, particularly given the person's age or stage of illness."[135]

Like parents making research decisions for children, surrogates labor under a heavy burden of responsibility. They are most concerned about the patient's current well-being and look to patients themselves to determine how to proceed. But surrogates and prospective subjects seem to have an easier time collaborating than do parents and children facing research decisions, perhaps because they were once equals.

WHERE TO GO FROM HERE

This look at the experiences of healthy volunteers, patient-subjects, and decision-makers for children and incapable adults reveals details often missing from standard analyses of research ethics and oversight. And the material I have presented here merely skims the surface. Research ethicists and policymakers have much more to learn about research subjects' perspectives.

Conventional approaches to medical ethics and research ethics share similar deficits. Professional narcissism and myopia have led traditional experts, including ethicists, to focus on abstract concepts, overlooking day-to-day interactions of subjects and researchers. Neither subjects' knowledge nor their ethical judgments have a place in these approaches. Research policies and principles of research ethics are removed from the realities of participation.

To maintain an ethical and effective subject protection system, we must hear from the people we are trying to protect. Ethical and policy deliberations should include people who know what it is like to participate in research. Input from subjects and surrogate decision-makers could help ethicists and officials devise more defensible and effective human research protections. Individuals with research experience should be regarded as experts whose knowledge and opinions are as valuable as the knowledge and opinions of professionals and scholars engaged in ethics and oversight work.

People with personal research experience should serve as members of institutional review boards (IRBs) evaluating proposed human studies. They should be recruited to advise IRBs on specific research questions too. Community-engaged and participatory research should enlist experienced subjects in study planning and execution as well. People with research experience should also be included in policy deliberations about specific research matters, such as the proper approach to securing informed consent to study participation. In later chapters, I describe how to make these changes.

NOTES

1. Larry Churchill, Joseph Fanning and David Schenk, *What Patients Teach: The Everyday Ethics of Health Care* (New York: Oxford University Press, 2013), 33, 137, 147. Perhaps reflecting differences between the two professions, codes developed by and for nurses are more attentive to patients' perspectives than are physician codes of ethics.
2. Ibid., 137.
3. Ibid., 147.
4. Michelle Eder et al., "Improving Informed Consent: Suggestions from Parents of Children with Leukemia," *Pediatrics* 119 (2007): e849–59, e850. One group commented on the dearth of information about patients' views of research decision-making, observing that most existing studies used questionnaires that failed to elicit patients' independent perspectives. C. Behrendt et al., "What Do Our Patients Understand about Their Trial Participation? Assessing Patients' Understanding of Their Informed Consent Consultation about Randomized Clinical Trials," *Journal of Medical Ethics* 37 (2011): 74–80.
5. Soren Madsen, S. Holm, and P. Riis, "Participating in a Clinical Trial? The Balancing of Options in the Loneliness of Autonomy: A Grounded Interview Study," *Acta Oncologica* 46 (2007): 49–59.
6. Karen Cox, "Enhancing Cancer Clinical Trial Management: Recommendations from a Qualitative Study of Trial Participants' Experiences," *Psycho-Oncology* 9 (2000): 314–22.
7. Madsen, Holm, and Riis, "Participating in a Clinical Trial?"
8. Claire Snowden, Jo Garcia, and Diana Elbourne, "Making Sense of Randomization: Responses of Parents of Critically

Ill Babies to Random Allocation of Treatment in a Clinical Trial," *Social Science and Medicine* 45 (1997): 1337–55.

9. For evidence that financial rewards are strong motivators for research participation, see Kirsten Bell and Amy Salmon, "What Women Who Use Drugs Have to Say about Ethical Research: Findings of an Exploratory Qualitative Study," *Journal of Empirical Research on Human Research Ethics* 6, no. 4 (2011): 84–98; Carmen Breitkopf et al., "Perceptions of Reimbursement for Clinical Trial Participation," *Journal of Empirical Research on Human Research Ethics* 6, no. 3 (2011): 31–38; Leanne Stunkel and Christine Grady, "More than the Money: A Review of the Literature Examining Healthy Volunteer Motivations," *Contemporary Clinical Trials* 32 (2011): 342–52; R. Hermann et al., "Adverse Events and Discomfort in Studies on Healthy Subjects: The Volunteer's Perspective," *European Journal of Clinical Pharmacology* 53 (2007): 207–14. Although subjects classify payment as a research benefit, the US Food and Drug Administration rejects this view. An agency document says, "Payment to research subjects is not considered a benefit, it is a recruitment incentive." US Food and Drug Administration, "Payment to Research Subjects—Information Sheet" (June 25, 2014). Retrieved March 25, 2015, from http://www.fda.gov/regulatoryinformation/guidances/ucm126429.htm.

10. One volunteer told a reporter that he rated studies according to the cash per study day that participants would receive; for example, he said that a study paying five hundred dollars for four weekends was "terrible." Barbara Solow, "The Secret Lives of Guinea Pigs," *Independent Weekly*, February 9, 2000. Retrieved March 25, 2015, from http://www.indyweek.com/gyrobase/Content?oid=13968.

11. See Carl Elliott, "Guinea-Pigging," *New Yorker*, January 7, 2008, 36, 40. In other interviews, a woman complained that since researchers are "getting paid to do the fucking research," subjects should "get paid to give them what they want!" Bell and Salmon, "What Women Who Use Drugs," 90.

12. See Elliott, "Guinea-Pigging," 40.

13. See Stunkel and Grady, "More than the Money."

14. Ibid. In one interview study, some healthy people portrayed volunteering as a form of wellness activity that allowed them to learn more about their current health and ways to maintain it. Susan Cox and Michael McDonald, "Ethics Is for Human Subjects Too: Participant Perspectives on Subject Responsibility," *Social Science and Medicine* 98 (2013): 224–31.

15. One volunteer told a journalist: "I've worked as an electrician and seen guys get electrocuted. Being a lab rat is the only work situation where you've got round-the-clock medical attention. It's the safest job I've ever been in." Josh McHugh, "Drug Test Cowboys: The Secret World of Pharmaceutical Trial Subjects," *Wired*, April 24, 2007. Retrieved March 25, 2015, from http://www.wired.com/wired/archive/15.05/feat_drugtest.html. A medical student seeking extra cash deemed trial participation "considerably more interesting than a supermarket job." Kate Mandeville, "My Life as a Guinea Pig," *BMJ* 332 (2006): 735.

16. Hermann et al., "Adverse Events." Two researchers dubbed this curiosity-driven volunteering "field-tripping." Cox and McDonald, "Ethics Is for Human Subjects," 229.

17. Solow, "Secret Lives."

18. Bell and Salmon, "What Women Who Use Drugs."

19. Stunkel and Grady, "More than the Money."

20. Bell and Salmon, "What Women Who Use Drugs."

21. Stunkel and Grady, "More than the Money."

22. "22 Nights and 23 Days: Diary of #1J, Drug Study Subject," 2006. Retrieved March 25, 2015, from http://www.guineapig-zero.com/23days.html.

23. Bell and Salmon, "What Women Who Use Drugs," 88.

24. Donno, "Awake with a Vengeance," in *Guinea Pig Zero: An Anthology of the Journal for Human Research Subjects*, ed. Robert Helms (New Orleans: Garrett County Press, 2002), 22–27, 26. Another volunteer wrote that "going to the cafeteria was something I lived for." Theresa Dulce, "Spanish Fly Guinea Pig: PPD Pharmaco, Where Slackers Refuel," in Helms, *Guinea Pig Zero*, 34–38, 36.

25. For a description of how researchers can apply the ethical principles of respect for persons, beneficence, and justice in routine interactions with prospective subjects, see Maria

Gyure et al., "Practical Considerations for Implementing Research Recruitment Etiquette," *IRB: Ethics & Human Research* 36, no. 6 (2014): 7–12.

26. After conducting an in-depth study of subjects' experiences, three analysts suggested that the term "impact" is a better way to refer to study burdens than the standard term "risk." Michael McDonald, Susan Cox, and Anne Townsend, "Toward Human Research Protection That Is Evidence-Based and Participant-Centered," in *Human Subjects Research Regulation: Perspectives on the Future*, ed. I. Glenn Cohen and Holly Fernandez Lynch (Cambridge, MA: MIT Press, 2014), 127–38.

27. Alison Motluk, "Diary of a Lab Rat," *New Scientist*, December 8, 2007, 38–41.

28. See Public Responsibility in Medicine & Research, "In Their Own Voices: A Discussion with Research Subjects Who Also Work in the Field of Subject Protections," 2010 Advancing Ethical Research Conference Proceedings. Retrieved March 6, 2015, from https://www.conferencepassport.com/index.asp.

29. Alex O'Meara, *Chasing Medical Miracles: The Promise and Peril of Clinical Trials* (New York: Walter, 2009), 115, citing Mikita Brottman, *I Was a Brain Slave*. Retrieved March 25, 2015, from http://www.guineapigzero.com/brainslave.html.

30. See subjects' comments in Margaret Russell et al., "Paying Research Subjects: Participants' Perspectives," *Journal of Medical Ethics* 26 (2000): 126–30, 127–28. Participants in a different study "focused on the time involved and various aspects of the study procedures . . ., including physical and emotional aspects of participation." They also noted time away from work, travel time, and time performing study-related procedures at home. Breitkopf et al., "Perceptions of Reimbursement," 34.

31. See women subjects' comments about a study that included gynecological examinations and an abstinence requirement in Breitkopf et al., "Perceptions of Reimbursement," 34.

32. Roberto Abadie, *The Professional Guinea Pig: Big Pharma and the Risky World of Human Subjects* (Durham, NC: Duke University Press, 2010), 57.

33. See Public Responsibility in Medicine & Research, "In Their Own Voices."

34. Dulce, "Spanish Fly Guinea Pig," 35.

35. Abadie, *Professional Guinea Pig*, 2–3.

36. In one survey of research subjects, "environmental study conditions appeared to have the most relevant impact on [subjects'] personal well-being." Hermann et al., "Adverse Events," 210.

37. Bell and Salmon, "What Women Who Use Drugs," 88.

38. Abadie, *Professional Guinea Pig*, 48 (quoting repeat volunteer Richard Helms).

39. Lisa McElroy, "The Anxious & the Damned," in Helms, *Guinea Pig Zero*, 18–21, 20. Another subject said her major problem was that "the study was so relaxed that I often didn't know whom I'd be seeing and they often didn't know if I was even scheduled for an interview." "22 Nights and 23 Days."

40. See Stunkel and Grady, "More than the Money"; Hermann et al., "Adverse Events," 21.

41. Rebecca Meiser, "Guinea Pig Gang," *Cleveland Scene*, March 22, 2006. Retrieved March 25, 2015, from http://www.clevescene.com/gyrobase/guinea-pig-gang/Content?oid=1494231.

42. Caitlin Kennedy et al., "When a Serious Adverse Event in Research Occurs, How Do Other Volunteers React?," *Journal of Empirical Research on Human Research Ethics* 6, no. 2 (2011): 47–56.

43. Abadie, *Professional Guinea Pig*, 36.

44. Elliott, "Guinea-Pigging," 41. When pharmacy students were asked whether they would enroll in hypothetical studies presenting different risk levels, students said that high payment would increase their willingness to enroll in a high-risk study. J. Bentley and P. Thacker, "The Influence of Risk and Monetary Payment on the Research Participation Decision Making Process," *Journal of Medical Ethics* 30 (2004): 294–98.

45. See National Institutes of Health, Office of Human Research Protections, "When Does Compensating Subjects Undermine Informed Consent or Parental Permission?" (October 18; 2013). Retrieved March 25, 2015, from http://www.hhs.gov/ohrp/policy/faq/informed-consent/when-does-compensating-subjects-undermine-informed-consent.html.

46. See Cynthia Cryder et al., "Informative Inducement: Study Payment as a Signal of Risk," *Social Science and Medicine* 70 (2010): 455–64.

47. Breitkopf et al., "Perceptions of Reimbursement," 34.
48. M. J. Czarny et al., "Payment to Healthy Volunteers in Clinical Research: The Research Subject's Perspective," *Clinical Pharmacology and Therapeutics* 87 (2010): 286–93.
49. Tony Truong et al., "Altruism among Participants in Cancer Clinical Trials," *Clinical Trials* 8 (2011): 616–23, 622.
50. Rebecca Pentz et al., "Therapeutic Misconception, Misestimation, and Optimism in Participants Enrolled in Phase I Trials," *Cancer* 118 (2012): 4571–78. Participants in early-stage cancer trials rarely receive a direct medical benefit.
51. Cox, "Enhancing Cancer Clinical Trial," 316.
52. Ricki Carroll et al., "Motivations of Patients with Pulmonary Arterial Hypertension to Participate in Randomized Controlled Trials," *Clinical Trials* 9 (2012): 348–57, 351.
53. Ann Cook and Helena Hoas, "Trading Places: What the Research Participant Can Tell the Investigator about Informed Consent," *Journal of Clinical and Research Bioethics* 2, no. 8 (2011): 1–7, 4. Another interview study found that most subjects sought access to medications, healthcare, and health monitoring tools. Anne Townsend and Susan Cox, "Accessing Health Services through the Back Door: A Qualitative Interview Study Investigating Reasons Why People Participate in Health Research in Canada," *BMC Medical Ethics* 14 (2013): 40–51.
54. Carroll et al., "Motivations of Patients," 353. One subject portrayed study tests as "free care." Ibid., 351.
55. Ibid., 353.
56. A large survey found that most subjects wanted to receive information about study results. Rhonda Kost et al., "Assessing Participant-Centered Outcomes to Improve Clinical Research," *New England Journal of Medicine* 369 (2013): 2179–81. Another group found that older children participating in cancer trials, as well as parents, believed they had a "strong right" to research results. Conrad Fernandez et al., "Providing Research Results to Participants: Attitudes and Needs of Adolescents and Parents of Children with Cancer," *Journal of Clinical Oncology* 27 (2009): 878–83.

57. Truong et al., "Altruism among Participants," 622. A recent survey of participants in research conducted at academic institutions produced somewhat different findings: the largest number of patient-subjects chose helping others as the most important factor motivating their participation, with "concern about the topic," "to find out more about my disease," and "to gain access to new treatment" as the next most important factors. It is possible that certain features of the study, such as a low survey return rate (29 percent of survey recipients) and the fact that survey respondents had participated in studies at leading medical centers rather than in other study settings, contributed to the "altruism-first" findings. See Kost et al., "Assessing Participant-Centered Outcomes."

58. Truong "Altruism among Participants," 622.

59. Cox, "Enhancing Cancer Clinical Trial," 316. A physician diagnosed with cancer criticized use of the term "eligibility" in connection with clinical trials because it suggests to patients that experimental treatment is special and desirable. Jane Poulson, "Bitter Pills to Swallow," *New England Journal of Medicine* 338 (1998): 1844–46.

60. Abadie, *Professional Guinea Pig*, 119.

61. One patient described participation as "It's almost me saying, 'What can I do to help you?'" Jonathan Kimmelman et al., "Consent for Nondiagnostic Research Biopsies: A Pilot Study of Participant Recall and Therapeutic Orientation," *IRB: Ethics & Human Research* 36, no. 3 (2014): 9–15.

62. The classic article on this topic is Benjamin Freedman, "Equipoise and the Ethics of Clinical Research," *New England Journal of Medicine* 317 (1987): 141–45.

63. See Madsen, Holm, and Riis, "Participating in a Clinical Trial?," in which almost all cancer patients considering trial participation doubted that treatments were in genuine equipoise and instead developed a preference for one treatment.

64. One cancer patient who did not get assigned to experimental intervention felt she had "lost the drawing of lots." Ibid., 56.

65. Katie Featherstone and Jenny Donovan, "'Why Don't They Just Tell Me Straight; Why Allocate It?' The Struggle to Make Sense of Participating in a Randomized Controlled Trial,"

Social Science and Medicine 55 (2002): 709–19, 713–14, 715, 717. See also Julie Brintnall-Karabelas et al., "Improving Recruitment in Clinical Trials: Why Eligible Participants Decline," *Journal of Empirical Research on Human Research Ethics* 6, no. 1 (2011): 69–74, in which individuals eligible for studies declined trial participation because they preferred to receive standard medical care.

66. Madsen, Holm, and Riis, "Participating in a Clinical Trial?," 56.

67. Ibid., 55. Much of the general public appears to share the discomfort with randomization. For example, in a questionnaire and interview study of adults in college classes, about half said they were "loathe [*sic*] to accept that a doctor might genuinely not know what treatment is best." About half also said it was unacceptable for a doctor to propose using randomization as a way to decide among treatments. They "assumed that just as much knowledge would be gained about which treatment is better if patients and doctors chose their treatment, rather than if treatments were allocated at random." Elizabeth Robinson et al., "Lay Conceptions of the Ethical and Scientific Justifications for Random Allocation in Clinical Trials," *Social Science and Medicine* 58 (2004): 811–24, 821.

68. See Christopher Daugherty et al., "Ethical, Scientific, and Regulatory Perspectives Regarding the Use of Placebos in Cancer Clinical Trials," *Journal of Clinical Oncology* 26 (2008): 1371–78.

69. In one study, patients said they would be disappointed and upset if they were assigned to placebo: "They did not acknowledge or value any possible placebo effect or the chance to avoid the potential risks of the real operation." Teresa Swift, "Sham Surgery Trial Controls: Perspectives of Patients and Their Relatives," *Journal of Empirical Research on Human Research Ethics* 7, no. 3 (2012): 15–28. In a survey of patient-subjects, 29 percent said that their top worry was being assigned to receive a placebo. D. McDonald and M. Lamberti, "The Psychology of Clinical Trials: Understanding Physician Motivation and Patient Perception," *Centerwatch Research Brief,* October 4, 2006. Retrieved April 19, 2015, from http://www.centerwatch.com/news-online/article/566/

the-psychology-of-clinical-trials-understanding-physician-motivation-and-patient-perception.

70. Swift, "Sham Surgery," 22.

71. Carroll et al., "Motivations of Patients," 352.

72. Madsen, Holm, and Riis, "Participating in a Clinical Trial?," 55, 57.

73. A reporter described the situation as follows: "It is one of the worst times imaginable—a cancer diagnosis, all the terror that goes with it, and then, sitting in a doctor's office and being asked to make a difficult decision about treatment. Then add questions about joining a trial." Gina Kolata, "Lack of Study Volunteers Hobbles Cancer Fight," *New York Times*, August 3, 2009. One group reported that breast cancer trial participants "were preoccupied with their diagnosis and treatment" during study discussions. Kimmelman et al., "Consent for Nondiagnostic Research," 14. Another group observed that cancer patients were "tired, impatient and distracted" when trial information was being discussed. Behrendt et al., "What Do Our Patients Understand," 78.

74. Madsen, Holm, and Riis, "Participating in a Clinical Trial?," 53. See Rebecca Dresser, "Volunteering for Research," in *Malignant: Medical Ethicists Confront Cancer*, ed. Rebecca Dresser (New York: Oxford University Press, 2012), 70–85.

75. Peter Korn, "Clinical Trials Stymied as Patients Balk at 'Experiments,'" *Portland Tribune*, January 16, 2014. Retrieved April 15, 2015, from http://portlandtribune.com/pt/9-news/207447-63461-clinical-trials-stymied-as-patients-balk-at-experiments.

76. Margaret Anderson, "Why Patients Turn Down Clinical Trials," *New York Times*, August 7, 2009.

77. Carroll et al., "Motivations of Patients."

78. Brintnall-Karabelas et al., "Improving Recruitment," 70. A survey of patient-subjects found that 31 percent were interested in public transportation to research facilities and 21 percent in having the least possible number of visits. McDonald and Lamberti, "Psychology of Clinical Trials."

79. See Robert Klitzman, *The Ethics Police? The Struggle to Make Human Research Safe* (New York: Oxford University Press, 2015), 95–99; O'Meara, *Chasing Medical Miracles*, 11–13; Ana

Iltis, "Costs to Subjects for Research Participation and the Informed Consent Process," *IRB: Ethics & Human Research* 26, no. 6 (2004): 9–13.

80. Iris Groeneveld et al., "Factors Associated with Non-participation and Drop-Out in a Lifestyle Intervention for Workers with an Elevated Risk of Cardovascular Disease," *International Journal of Behavioral Nutrition and Physical Activity* 6 (2009): 80–89.

81. McDonald et al., "Toward Human Research Protection," 130.

82. Cook and Hoas, "Trading Places," 5.

83. C. Daniel Mullins et al., "Patient-Centeredness in the Design of Clinical Trials," *Value in Health* 17 (2014): 471–76.

84. Cox, "Enhancing Cancer Clinical Trial," 317.

85. Ann Cook, Helena Hoas, and Jane Joyner, "The Protector and the Protected: What Regulators and Researchers Can Learn from IRB Members and Subjects," *Narrative Inquiry in Bioethics* 3 (2013): 51–65, 62. Another team said that most of the cancer patients they interviewed "expressed doubts about industrial financing of trials owing to worries about industry placing commercial motives before the interests of patients." Soren Madsen, S. Holm, and P. Riis, "Attitudes towards Clinical Research among Cancer Trial Participants: An Interview Study Using a Grounded Theory Approach," *Journal of Medical Ethics* 33 (2007): 234–40, 236–37.

86. Cook, Hoas, and Joyner, "The Protector and the Protected," 61.

87. Cook and Hoas, "Trading Places," 5.

88. Ibid.

89. Kost et al., "Assessing Participant-Centered Outcomes," 2180.

90. Cook, Hoas, and Joyner, "The Protector and the Protected," 55.

91. See Gail Henderson et al., "Clinical Trials and Medical Care: Defining the Therapeutic Misconception," *PLoS Medicine* 4 (2007): e324.

92. Cancer trial participants' responses to one survey suggested that many failed to understand that the trials' purpose was to benefit future patients. Many also didn't understand that study treatments had not been shown to be the best treatment for their cancer. Steven Joffe et al., "Quality of Informed Consent in Cancer Clinical Trials: A Cross-Sectional Survey," *Lancet* 358 (2001): 1772–77.

93. Ibid., 1774. In an interesting twist, experienced subjects in a different interview study understood that research offered uncertain medical benefit but said benefits from standard medical care were similarly uncertain. Townsend and Cox, "Accessing Health Services," 48.

94. For example, in a survey of cancer trial participants, many thought they had a better-than-average chance of experiencing health benefit from the investigational drugs they were taking, despite understanding that the purpose of the trials was to help future patients rather than trial participants. Lynn Jansen et al., "Unrealistic Optimism in Early-Phase Oncology Trials," IRB: Ethics & Human Research 33, no. 1 (2011): 1–8.

95. Ibid.; Don Swekowski and Deborah Barnbaum, "The Gambler's Fallacy, the Therapeutic Misconception, and Unrealistic Optimism," IRB: Ethics & Human Research 35, no. 2 (2013): 1–6.

96. Joshua Crites and Eric Kodish, "Unrealistic Optimism and the Ethics of Phase I Cancer Research," Journal of Medical Ethics 39 (2013): 403–6.

97. Pentz et al., "Therapeutic Misconception," 4575–76. See also Scott Kim et al., "Research Participants' 'Irrational' Expectations: Common or Commonly Mismeasured?," IRB: Ethics & Human Research 35, no. 1 (2013): 1–9, which discusses other factors that can lead subjects to express optimism about personal benefit.

98. Daniel Sulmasy et al., "The Culture of Faith and Hope: Patients' Justifications for Their High Estimations of Expected Therapeutic Benefit When Enrolling in Early Phase Oncology Trials," Cancer 116 (2010): 3702–11, 3707.

99. Pentz et al., "Therapeutic Misconception," 4575. This study of cancer trial participants also found a subgroup the authors called "therapeutic pessimists," who believed they had a lower chance of benefit or higher risk of harm than others enrolled in the trials.

100. Cook, Hoas, and Joyner, "The Protector and the Protected," 57.

101. Ibid., 55–57.

102. Cook and Hoas, "Trading Places," 3. See also Kimmelman et al., "Consent for Nondiagnostic Resarch," 13, which found

that many patients' choice to participate in a trial reflected their trust in the research institution and investigators.

103. Cox, "Enhancing Cancer Clinical Trial," 316.

104. Madsen, Holm, and Riis, "Participating in a Clinical Trial?," 54.

105. Ibid., 55. In another interview study, one-third of patients said they preferred that the doctor decide about trial enrollment. Carroll et al., "Motivations of Patients," 348.

106. Valerie Shilling and Bridget Young, "How Do Parents Experience Being Asked to Enter a Child in a Randomised Controlled Trial?," *BMC Medical Ethics* 10 (2009): 1–11, 2.

107. Patrina Caldwell et al., "Parents' Attitudes toward Children's Participation in Randomized Controlled Trials," *Journal of Pediatrics* 142 (2003): 554–59.

108. Shilling and Young, "How Do Parents," 2.

109. Ibid., 5.

110. Jeremy Vanhelst et al., "Effect of Child Health Status on Parents' Allowing Children to Participate in Pediatric Research," *BMC Medical Ethics* 14 (2013): 7–16. For a review of the evidence on parents' views of their children's research participation, see Shilling and Young, "How Do Parents."

111. See Shilling and Young, "How Do Parents," 7, which notes that some parents might cite altruism to justify their decision to enroll children or to portray that decision in socially positive terms.

112. Public Responsibility in Medicine and Research, "In Our Own Voices: Pediatric and Adolescent Research Subjects Share Their Stories," Annual Human Research Protection Programs Conference, December 2, 2007. Retrieved April 20, 2015, from http://www.meetingproceedings.us/2007/primr/contents/audio/web/81973/player.html.

113. Eric Kodish et al., "Communication of Randomization in Childhood Leukemia Trials," *Journal of the American Medical Association* 291 (2004): 470–75. According to another study team, parents "are vulnerable both to misunderstanding the distinction between research and treatment and to misunderstanding and overestimating the potential of medical research to benefit their children." Rebecca Schaffer et al., "Parents' Online Portrayals of Pediatric Treatment

and Research Options," *Journal of Empirical Research on Human Research Ethics* 4, no. 3 (2009): 73–87, 81.

114. Snowden, Garcia, and Elbourne, "Making Sense of Randomization," 1345.

115. Public Responsibility in Medicine and Research, "Living Room Conversation: A Discussion with Research Subjects and Their Advocates," Advancing Ethical Research Conference, November 2009. Retrieved April 20, 2015, from http://www.meetingproceedings.com/2009/aerc/contents/index.asp.

116. Shilling and Young, "How Do Parents," 4.

117. Kerry Woolfall et al., "Parents' Agendas in Paediatric Clinical Trial Recruitment Are Different from Researchers' and Often Remain Unvoiced: A Qualitative Study," *PLoS One* 7 (2013): e67352.

118. Public Responsibility in Medicine and Research, "In Our Own Voices."

119. Shilling and Young, "How Do Parents," 3.

120. Ibid., 3.

121. See Ulrica Swartling et al., "'My Parents Decide If I Can. I Decide If I Want To.' Children's Views on Participation in Medical Research," *Journal of Empirical Research on Human Subjects Research* 6, no. 4 (2011): 68–75; Yoram Unguru, Anne Sill, and Naynesh Kamani, "Experiences of Children Enrolled in Pediatric Oncology Research: Implications for Assent," *Pediatrics* 125 (2010): e876–83.

122. Public Responsibility in Medicine and Research, "In Our Own Voices."

123. David Wendler and Tammara Jenkins, "Children and Their Parents' Views on Facing Research Risks," *Archives of Pediatric & Adolescent Medicine* 162 (2008): 9–14.

124. Shilling and Young, "How Do Parents," 8.

125. Unguru, Sill, and Kamani, "Experiences of Children," e880.

126. Betty Black, Malory Wechsler, and Linda Fogarty, "Decision Making for Participation in Dementia Research," *American Journal of Geriatric Psychiatry* 21 (2013): 355–63, 359.

127. Jason Karlawish et al., "The Views of Alzheimer Disease Patients and Their Study Partners on Proxy Consent for Clinical Trial Enrollment," *American Journal of Geriatric Psychiatry* 16 (2008): 240–47, 244.

128. Laura Dunn et al., "'Thinking about It for Somebody Else': Alzheimer's Disease Research and Proxy Decision Makers' Translation of Ethical Principles into Practice," *American Journal of Geriatric Psychiatry* 21 (2013): 337–45, 343.

129. Ibid., 341.

130. Karlawish et al., "Views of Alzheimer." In a third inquiry, researchers found that 42 percent of surrogates favored the best-interests standard and 20 percent favored a combination of the best-interests and substituted-judgment standards. Just 9 percent favored the substituted-judgment standard. Black, Wechsler, and Fogarty, "Decision Making for Participation," 361.

131. Dunn et al., "'Thinking about It,'" 343.

132. Karlawish et al., "Views of Alzheimer," 245.

133. Dunn et al., "'Thinking about It,'" 342.

134. Ibid.

135. Ibid., 343.

4

The Hidden World of Subjects

Rule-Breaking in Clinical Trials

■□■

IN 2015, the *New England Journal of Medicine* published the results of an HIV prevention trial involving more than five thousand women in sub-Saharan Africa. Women enrolled in the trial were randomly assigned to receive different combinations of pills, vaginal gels, and placebos. According to the trial findings, none of the drug regimens reduced the rates of HIV infection.[1]

Researchers had a startling explanation for the findings. Rather than being evidence that the drugs were ineffective, the findings indicated that trial subjects had failed to use the pills and gels as directed. During the trial, women claimed they were following the study requirements for drug use, returning empty medication containers as proof. But blood tests revealed that many women supposedly taking active medication had low levels of the study drugs in their bodies.

An earlier version of this chapter was published as "Subversive Subjects: Rule-Breaking and Deception in Clinical Trials," *Journal of Law, Medicine and Ethics* 41 (2013): 829–40.

The researchers later learned that many women had actually discarded the study products.

Researchers traced this behavior to the women's worries about drug safety. Other contributing factors were fear that their medication use would lead others to think they had HIV, a stigmatizing condition, and lack of trust in the researchers. However, the women wanted to continue receiving the payments and medical benefits that went along with study participation.[2] To prevent similar problems in the future, trial investigators advised other researchers to adopt "measures of adherence that do not rely solely on self-reporting and that are not easily manipulated by participants."[3]

According to a *New York Times* report, this incident "opened an ethical debate about how to run [HIV prevention] studies in poor countries."[4] But that description is too narrow. Subjects in many countries and many types of studies engage in the same sort of covert rule-breaking seen in the HIV prevention trial. One US drug researcher called this rule-breaking "the crazy uncle in the attic that nobody likes to talk about."[5] Although scientific reports on research rarely acknowledge it, "nonadherence"[6] is a major problem in drug and other clinical trials.

When their personal interests conflict with study demands, some subjects surreptitiously break the rules. Although they don't necessarily intend to compromise the quality of research, they do. Like researchers who secretly influence subject assignment in randomized clinical trials,[7] rule-breaking subjects elevate their own desires and concerns above the trial requirements that are applied to produce good data.

Both subjects themselves and the journalists and scholars who write about them have described concealed rule-breaking by healthy volunteers and patients enrolled in studies. Researchers have also reported uncovering some of the rule-breaking. But because relatively few studies adopt measures to detect this behavior, it often goes unnoticed. Researchers tend to focus on study design and results, "viewing adherence as a nuisance and a somewhat tangential concern."[8] They overestimate subjects' adherence to trial rules, "often assum[ing] that medications are taken correctly."[9]

Even researchers who look for rule-breaking don't detect all of it. Some rule-breaking is, as a practical matter, undetectable. Researchers often have no option other than to rely on subjects' accounts of their health histories and compliance with trial requirements. In some situations, independent verification is impossible. In others, verification would require researchers to adopt costly and intrusive monitoring procedures that few subjects would tolerate.

Although the full extent of rule-breaking is unknown, its existence is undeniable. Clinical trial subjects are not passive followers of researchers' orders; they are active agents living their own lives and promoting what they see as their own interests.[10] But in rejecting the constraints that research imposes, subjects diminish the value of research results.[11] They also create health risks for themselves and others.

Scholars and policymakers devote a great deal of attention to the ethical issues raised by so-called deception research—studies in which investigators deceive subjects to acquire otherwise unobtainable data.[12] But few consider the reverse situation, in which subjects deceive investigators to advance their own agendas. Deceptive subjects are a reality in clinical research, and their deception merits scrutiny too.[13]

From one vantage point, rule-breaking subjects behave unethically. Besides creating health risks, they ignore ethical responsibilities to observe research agreements and tell the truth. At the same time, rule-breaking subjects expose ethical problems with the design and conduct of clinical trials. Features of the research environment create fertile ground for subject rule-breaking. Researchers often turn to intensified policing and guidance strategies to reduce rule-breaking, but collaborative reforms are more consistent with the partnership model of clinical research.

EVIDENCE OF RULE-BREAKING

Healthy Volunteers in Phase 1 Studies

Evidence of rule-breaking in clinical trials comes from subjects' firsthand accounts, interviews with subjects, case reports, and empirical studies. Professional guinea pigs tell the most vivid stories. These individuals make at least part of their living from the payments they receive for participating in phase 1 trials evaluating the effects of investigational drugs in healthy people. Some have published essays about their experiences. From 1996 to 2008, a professional guinea pig named Robert Helms published *Guinea Pig Zero*, a print and online journal reporting on this group's research experiences.[14] A few academics have also written about professional guinea pigs.[15] Medical anthropologist Roberto Abadie's in-depth ethnography is a particularly rich account of how some members of this group perceive their "work."[16]

Volunteers who are focused on earning money through research participation adopt a variety of deceptive practices to gain admission to studies. One thing they lie about is past trial participation. Volunteers must wait at least thirty days after a phase 1 drug trial ends before enrolling in another one.[17] Mandatory waiting periods are based on the time it takes for drugs to be eliminated from the body. Researchers want to avoid drug interactions that can compromise data quality and put subjects at risk. But volunteers employ different strategies to avoid the wait. They seek out studies at new locations that have no record of their recent trial participation. To prepare for study screening tests, they "cleanse" their bodies by following certain diets and using substances like cranberry juice, water, goldenseal, marigold flowers, and other herbal remedies. They also take iron supplements to counter the effects of having had multiple blood samples taken in previous trials.[18]

Volunteers lie about other things in their quest for trial admission. Study eligibility requirements are designed to promote data quality and protect subjects from harm. Repeat volunteers know about these requirements and plan accordingly. Besides using the cleansing remedies described above, they supply false information about their use of alcohol, medication, recreational drugs, cigarettes, and caffeine. They also lie about their ages, medical histories, dietary practices, and exercise habits. Some participate in more than one trial at the same time, which is usually not permitted.[19]

The deception doesn't end once volunteers gain admission to trials. Subjects are told that to earn full compensation, they must conform to study requirements. But study participation can demand a lot of subjects. Some chafe against the restrictions and devise ways to evade them without being detected. This sort of rule-breaking is easier to achieve in "outpatient" studies than in the on-site studies that require subjects to live at test facilities for days or weeks. But even volunteers in on-site trials (one subject called them "lockdowns"[20]) get away with some misbehavior.

Standardizing diet and environmental conditions is a way to increase the odds that test results are produced by study interventions instead of other factors. But to get around dietary requirements, subjects have smuggled prohibited food into facilities and broken into locked pantries for forbidden treats. Although meals are monitored in onsite trials, subjects say they hide and later discard the unappetizing food they are supposed to eat. Phase 1 drug trials often exclude vegetarians, but some gain admission by concealing this information. Once in the trial, they maintain their diet by trading meat for other subjects' vegetables.[21] There are also reports of subjects drinking alcohol and taking illegal drugs during trials.[22]

Volunteers disregard rules about medication use too. Subjects who concealed their medication history to gain trial admission find ways to continue taking prohibited medications.[23] Volunteers in off-site trials don't always take their study drugs as directed, and even subjects in on-site trials are at times able to discard pills.[24] Participants sometimes fail to report symptoms that could be related to study drugs, because they fear they will be removed from the study for health reasons.[25]

Professional guinea pigs portray these actions as reasonable responses to researchers' unrealistic expectations. As one trial subject put it, "The perfect volunteer they require doesn't exist. Everybody lies about complying. I lied about my family medical history, yeah, about drug use, taking medicine."[26] Experienced volunteers know that truthful answers could result in their exclusion from studies and loss of the payments they hope to receive. They also doubt the value and quality of studies for drug companies and in turn feel little obligation to play by drug study rules.

Patient-Subjects in Clinical Trials

By their own admission, the repeat volunteers who populate the world of phase 1 drug testing fabricate and conceal information about past trial experience, medical history, adherence to trial requirements, and intentions to cooperate with those requirements. But rule-breaking is not limited to these volunteers. Rule-breaking also occurs in the later-phase studies that evaluate the effects of drugs and other interventions in patients. The evidence here comes primarily from empirical studies of subjects' nonadherence. Case reports and interviews supply additional evidence of nonadherence in later-phase trials.

Research sponsors typically don't pay patients for participation in later-phase trials. The customary view is that potential health benefits to patients substitute for the financial rewards offered to healthy volunteers. This view is changing, however, and some trials now offer relatively large payments to patient-subjects. Like healthy volunteers, patient-subjects who are focused on financial rewards sometimes falsify information related to their trial eligibility and conceal this deception after they are admitted.[27]

More often, it is the potential medical benefit offered by later-phase trials that creates an incentive for patient-subjects to lie. Many people coping with debilitating or life-threatening illnesses enter trials with the goal of improving their health. If trial requirements interfere with this goal, some subjects disregard those requirements and conceal their rule-breaking from the research team. A desire to please researchers also leads subjects to exaggerate their adherence.[28]

Although subject rule-breaking in later-phase trials often goes unnoticed, some investigators take measures to detect it. These measures allow researchers to compare subjects' reports about their study behavior with objective indications of that behavior. In one example, investigators in an asthma study gave subjects inhalers that (unbeknownst to the subjects) were equipped to record the dates and times that medication was released. Almost one-third of the subjects "dumped" all or most of the medication at least once before meeting with study staff, revealing their failure to use the inhalers as directed. Those subjects withheld this information from the researchers.[29] In another study, the pill containers that subjects returned to researchers indicated that 92 percent of subjects were taking the study drug as directed, but blood tests revealed that only 70 percent of subjects had actually done so.[30]

Rule-breaking can be a particular problem in later-phase trials comparing investigational drugs with drugs already in medical use. Patients entering trials are often dissatisfied with their current treatments and hope they will be assigned to receive a new and potentially better one. They don't want to be assigned to control groups receiving standard treatment or a placebo.[31] And as one researcher put it, "people allocated to less desirable control conditions where they feel deprived of their preferred treatment . . . may lose heart, or act up."[32] This phenomenon is most likely to occur in nonblinded trials, but "even when participants do not know their treatment group, they often guess or suspect, correctly or incorrectly," which drugs they are receiving.[33]

Patients in this situation disregard a variety of research requirements. Some enter trials with the specific intent to drop out early if their symptoms don't improve within a certain time.[34] Some share drugs with other study subjects to ensure that each person receives at least some of the preferred one. During the early years of the HIV/AIDS epidemic, desperate patients admitted to both of these actions, as well as to "frequent cheating, even bribery, to gain entry to studies."[35] Researchers have observed similar behavior in other trials. So-called contamination occurs when "participants assigned to a control condition try to gain access to or adopt elements of the intervention condition."[36] For example, cancer survivors assigned to the control group in an exercise study were found to actually be exercising at the same level as the intervention group.[37]

According to one review, "Research demonstrates that many clinical trial participants are overestimating their adherence and not providing the study investigators with honest self-reports."[38] Estimates are that up to 30 percent of trial subjects fail to take study drugs as directed. One expert suggests that the rates could be even higher: "there is considerable anecdotal evidence, if not hard data, that most patient-subjects are not fully compliant."[39]

Subjects in Other Kinds of Studies

Rule-breaking isn't limited to drug and other treatment studies. Subjects in other kinds of research also report such behavior. For example, a journalist writing about his experience as a study participant revealed his own rule-breaking. The study he joined was designed to evaluate the effects of a "Stone Age" diet. As the study progressed, he grew weary of the monotonous diet he was expected to follow. When he lost weight, researchers wanted him to eat more. But he failed to comply. Instead, he "sneaked extra clothes onto the scale to avoid . . . the growing portions of pork and pineapple they heaped on my plate as my weight fell."[40]

Covert rule-breaking also creates problems in deception research. While deception is used most commonly in psychology research, it is used in clinical trials too. For example, studies of placebo effects in medicine often deceive subjects about study aims, and drug trials sometimes fail to inform subjects that they will all receive placebos during a baseline assessment period.[41]

The problems arise when subjects suspect that a study involves deception. Such awareness can affect subjects' responses, distorting study findings. In poststudy debriefings, researchers typically ask subjects whether they suspected they were being deceived. Using computerized questionnaires and other methods, researchers have discovered that some subjects don't admit to their suspicions when they are debriefed. In an ironic twist, subjects deceive the investigators who sought to deceive them. Deceptive subjects say they are concerned that a truthful answer will jeopardize their payment or course credit, get them into trouble, or upset the investigators.[42]

No one knows how many subjects fail to follow the rules, but it is clear that rule-breaking happens. To promote their personal interests, some subjects undermine the research enterprise. Some subjects freely admit to bad behavior, but others try to hide it. Although researchers discover some rule-breaking, an unknown amount remains undiscovered.

WHAT'S WRONG
WITH RULE-BREAKING

From a public health perspective, rule-breaking subjects present a serious threat. Their actions reduce the validity of trial results, with potentially harmful consequences to patients, as well as to subjects in later trials that rely on the inaccurate results. Rule-breaking subjects expose themselves to heightened research risks too. They also disregard ethical principles governing keeping promises and telling the truth.[43]

Distorted Study Findings

Subjects' rule-breaking can lead to inaccurate scientific conclusions about research interventions. For example, undetected nonadherence contributes to mistaken judgments about the safety and proper dosages of investigational drugs. When subjects discard study medications and conceal this action, researchers record a higher level of drug use than actually occurred. This information could lead them to conclude that a drug is safe and effective at the recorded rather than actual level of use—but the recorded dosage could be less safe than the lower amount to which subjects were actually exposed.[44] Similarly, when subjects fail to report symptoms that might be caused by an investigational drug, researchers may conclude that the drug is safer than it actually is.[45] And when subjects share study medications during trials, it becomes more difficult to detect both positive and negative effects of those medications.[46] According to some experts, many drugs have been approved at unnecessarily high dosages, only to eventually be lowered after "we overdosed a whole lot of patients."[47]

Subjects entering trials on false pretenses also jeopardize study findings. Researchers fooled into thinking that subjects were qualified for drug studies may attribute to a study drug effects that were actually caused by subjects' preexisting health conditions, exposure to alcohol, or other factors unrelated to the intervention. As a consequence, a "potentially useful medication [could be] discarded because of an adverse event falsely attributed to the drug."[48] When healthy people are mistakenly admitted into trials that are supposed to include only subjects with specific medical conditions, "any subjective reports of disease progression or remission would also be fictitious."[49]

Although methodological strategies aimed at reducing the impact of subject nonadherence exist, these strategies are imperfect. Researchers and regulators rely on two types of analysis in assessing a drug's safety and effectiveness. One type, called intent-to-treat analysis, includes data from all subjects initially enrolled in a study, including those who later withdrew. This approach supplies information about a drug's potential health impact, because a certain number of patients will also stop taking their drugs. The other approach includes data from only those subjects who completed the trial. This supplies information about the drug's effects in individuals exposed to the full drug regimen.[50] It is much easier to adjust an analysis when noncompliant subjects are detected and withdrawn from a study than when such subjects successfully conceal their behavior and remain in a study. Researchers cannot adjust an analysis to take into account behavior of which they are unaware.[51]

The bottom line is that covert rule-breaking reduces the accuracy of research findings. Inaccurate findings create risks to subjects enrolled in later studies that build on those findings as well as to patients taking drugs that were approved based on faulty data. Inaccurate findings can prematurely halt drug development too, depriving patients of potentially beneficial new drugs. More broadly, rule-breaking can have a negative impact whenever health recommendations rely on the flawed data that result from such behavior.

Risks to Self

Subjects concealing or fabricating information about their medical histories and prior trial experiences put themselves at risk too. Certain medical conditions and past drug exposures can increase a person's susceptibility to harm from trial interventions. In a few documented cases, concealing this information proved deadly to subjects.[52] For instance, a young woman in a National Institutes of Health study using healthy volunteers suffered a fatal cardiac arrest after concealing a history of previous cardiac arrest from the investigators.[53] Undoubtedly more common are less serious acute effects among subjects who withhold relevant health information. One research group reported that three volunteers experienced ill effects after failing to tell investigators about food allergies, diabetes, and cardiac abnormalities.[54] Possible long-term effects of inappropriate research exposures are another concern, especially for volunteers who participate repeatedly in phase 1 drug trials.[55]

It's sometimes argued that subjects should be free to decide whether to expose themselves to undue risk, but it's not clear that all deceptive subjects understand the risks they are taking. In one survey, for example, a few healthy volunteers admitted they did not realize that providing an inaccurate health history could elevate the risk of study participation.[56] Moreover, most people think that subjects should not be exposed to unreasonable research risks even if they consent to such risks.[57]

Ethical Violations

Besides risking harm to themselves and others, rule-breaking subjects fail to meet their moral responsibilities "to be truthful and to abide by the terms of participation."[58] When subjects consent to join studies, they consent to observe the study requirements. If participation proves too burdensome, they are free to withdraw. But subjects who remain in a study while violating its terms breach their research agreements. Patients entering studies with fixed plans to withdraw if they are assigned to an unwanted treatment group or if their condition doesn't improve also fail to meet their ethical responsibilities. Individuals who falsify or conceal information to gain admission to trials, and those who conceal their noncompliant behavior during trials, are engaging in unjustified deception.[59]

People are not entitled to manipulate the research system for personal gain. As ethicist John Arras put it, "no one has a duty to become a research subject in the first place, but by entering a protocol, subjects enter into a moral relationship with researchers by promising or 'contracting' to abide by certain restrictions for the benefits of participation."[60] Indeed, some professional guinea pigs share this view. Just Another Lab Rat, a website created by a repeat volunteer, lists five "Cardinal Rules for Volunteering for Clinical Research," all of which emphasize the volunteer's responsibility to comply with research requirements.[61]

In sum, it's easy to fault subjects for their rule-breaking. They risk harm to themselves and others, violate agreements, and deceive researchers. But rule-breaking subjects are not the only ones at fault. Some rule-breaking is the unsurprising side effect of a research system with ethical deficiencies.

HOW RESEARCH CONTRIBUTES TO RULE-BREAKING

We often hear about the essential contribution subjects make to the research endeavor. The literature is full of statements like the following: "Clinical investigators, research institutions, and funding agencies were indispensable to [the past century's medical] advances. Equally important were the millions of individuals who agreed to participate in the research that proved the effectiveness of the interventions that worked and, no less importantly, the ineffectiveness of those that did not."[62] But rule-breaking subjects expose a gap between the platitudes and the reality. These subjects present a different and less egalitarian vision of human research. In this vision, subjects' interests and contributions are devalued. They are treated with disrespect and discourtesy, regarded more as servants than as research partners. In turn, they feel little allegiance to the research mission.

Subjects trace their disillusionment to several kinds of mistreatment. Repeat trial volunteers complain about substandard conditions in some research units. They tell tales of poorly organized trials, inattentive staff, and silly rules like mandatory bedtimes in on-site studies. To call attention to problems like these, *Guinea Pig Zero's* publisher, Robert Helms, prepared "report cards" on different research units, assigning low grades for deficiencies like bad food and mediocre staff as well as excessive security, waiting times, tests, and follow-up visits.[63]

Helms's grades took into account the quality of the consent process as well. Helms and other study volunteers have described several problems in this area. Researchers explain studies poorly and are unprepared to answer subjects' questions. They make it difficult for subjects to get copies of study protocols, and they change consent forms after subjects have signed them.[64] Some subjects—including a well-known US bioethicist—report being told they were not allowed to withdraw from studies, a clear violation of the federal research regulations.[65]

Subjects complain that researchers are sometimes dishonest too. A website offering tips to volunteers reported that staff members at some research units inflated the number of subjects needed for trials, misleading individuals about their odds of being accepted. This strategy allows the staff to be highly selective about who is actually chosen, wasting the time of the other people who show up. Staff members also tell would-be volunteers that they have been admitted to trials when they are actually alternates who will be included only if others fail to show up.[66]

When subjects experience disrespectful treatment like this, relationships with researchers become adversarial. Professional guinea pigs use stark language to express their resentment. They present "images of torture, sex work, or prostitution when describing their activities."[67] They see themselves as "meat puppets" and "brain sluts."[68] One wrote of "sitting around like an animal in the zoo," with people observing her through windows and delivering food to her room.[69]

Subjects blame at least some of their rule-breaking on researchers' misbehavior. According to Roberto Abadie, professional guinea pigs use "everyday forms of resistance" to oppose "conditions that dehumanize, alienate, and exploit them."[70] This phenomenon is not limited to the professional volunteers—patient-subjects react negatively to unsatisfactory study conditions too. Nonadherence is more likely in studies involving unreasonable time demands, unfriendly staff, and unpleasant surroundings.[71]

At times, researchers are complicit in subjects' rule-breaking. According to Helms, "everyone," including the research staff, knows that guinea pigs lie to get into high-paying trials.[72] One volunteer wrote about a study director who told her that alcohol and certain medications were prohibited during the trial, then winked and said, "But hey, we're not always going to be looking over your shoulder."[73] Researchers who fail to take study requirements seriously are on thin ice when they complain about subjects who do the same thing.

Hostility and cynicism aren't the only detrimental psychological responses that can be fostered by the research environment. Nonadherent subjects who see researchers as authority figures may keep quiet out of a reluctance to let down or anger the team. According to one researcher, people appearing on paper as "super-compliers" are actually among the least compliant—it's just that "[t]hey are very nice people who don't want to disappoint you."[74] Similarly, subjects in deception research don't admit to suspecting the deception because "they are worried that they might ruin the study" and thus upset the investigator.[75] Researchers' power to remove subjects from studies is probably the biggest factor in concealed rule-breaking. Subjects hoping for full payment, medical benefit, or course credit have strong incentives to cover up their deviations from study requirements.

Researchers often portray subjects as equal partners in the research endeavor. But not every subject sees things this way. At least some believe their role is devalued and their agency overlooked. These subjects say they are too often treated as mere data sources whose personal needs and concerns get in the way of the research process. Others say they are ashamed or afraid to admit when they fall short of researchers' expectations. Subjects who see researchers as authority figures may respond in ways that damage the research mission.

RESPONSES TO RULE-BREAKING

People worried about rule-breaking subjects propose a variety of measures to address the problem. These encompass three general approaches: more vigilant policing of subjects' behavior; intensified efforts to guide subjects toward adherence; and increased collaboration with subjects to develop mutually acceptable research conditions.

Researchers attempting to reduce rule-breaking through better policing offer an array of strategies. One is to increase external monitoring of subjects. A variety of "assays, devices, tests, and biochemical measures" allow researchers to detect whether subjects comply with bans on smoking, alcohol, and recreational drugs.[76] With electronic monitoring devices such as the inhalers used in the asthma study I described earlier, researchers can determine subjects' true compliance rates. Experts predict that the future will bring more external monitoring tools. Scientists are developing "smart pills" with microchips that send a computer alert when the pill is swallowed.[77] Two analysts report that researchers and physicians "are on the threshold of having an armamentarium of 'big brother' strategies to determine who is noncompliant."[78]

Other policing strategies focus on enforcing trial eligibility criteria. To prevent repeat volunteers from violating waiting-period and other eligibility requirements, some countries, as well as a few US research institutions, have created centralized databases that store information about each study subject's medical and trial history. Researchers screening potential subjects for new trials can consult the database to determine a candidate's prior record and then reject the ones who are ineligible.[79]

Researchers also use screening measures to identify and exclude people who are unlikely to comply with study requirements. According to one review, "the best predictor of future adherence behavior is past adherence behavior."[80] Researchers assess adherence by conducting a brief preliminary study in which they evaluate a person's performance on tasks like returning phone calls and showing up for visits on time. Those who perform poorly are then excluded from the main study.[81]

Assessing short-term adherence is expensive, so researchers have tried to find simple demographic criteria that would allow them to separate probable rule breakers from rule followers. They haven't had much success, however. For example, researchers could find no significant differences between subjects who were and were not compliant in the previously described asthma study that used dose-detecting inhalers.[82]

Another policing strategy is to impose monetary penalties on subjects who fail to follow study rules or drop out "for apparently trivial nonmedical reasons."[83] Supporters of this approach say that research agreements should be regarded as contracts, and subjects should be legally responsible for fulfilling their side of the bargain. Although critics raise legal and practical questions about the usefulness of such an approach, defenders say it would deter subjects from misbehaving and send a strong message about the moral responsibilities of individuals enrolled in trials.[84]

Researchers favoring intensified guidance over policing believe that communication and persuasion are more ethical and effective ways to reduce rule-breaking.[85] On the assumption that rule-breaking is often due to ignorance or forgetfulness, experts urge researchers to distribute consent forms and informational handouts that clearly describe what subjects are expected to do. Other guidance techniques are designed to make adherence easier. Electronic diaries and cell phone alerts prompt subjects to take study medications. "Compliance packaging" for study drugs includes clear messages and graphics highlighting essential information about study drug regimens.[86]

Researchers adopt other guidance measures to "re-educate" subjects during trials. At one-on-one meetings and over the telephone they remind subjects of study requirements and subject responsibilities.[87] Subjects who miss appointments, appear unenthusiastic, or exhibit other behaviors suggesting they are "at risk" for noncompliance "become targets to work on."[88] According to one optimistic expert, "Once study participants understand why it is important for them to take the study medications as prescribed, they will feel 'safer' providing honest feedback to the study team."[89]

Policing and guidance strategies can be effective in detecting and deterring certain forms of rule-breaking, and they can be used in ethically acceptable ways. For example, external monitoring devices are acceptable when used with subjects' awareness and permission, rather than secretly as they were in the dose-detecting inhaler study. Although guidance and persuasion strategies can be patronizing and intrusive, this needn't be the case. Many subjects will welcome reminders, clear information, and other aids that help them reconcile the demands of research participation with the demands of ordinary life.

At bottom, however, policing and guidance strategies reinforce the research hierarchy. Communication and persuasion may be more collegial than policing, but both strategies treat subjects more as subordinates than as partners in the research endeavor.

The collaborative approach is a more respectful response, for it regards subjects as agents with their own legitimate concerns and values. Researchers adopting collaborative strategies recognize that features of the research system contribute to rule-breaking and deception. They also see punitive measures and moral censure as arrogant and often ineffective. From their perspective, rule-breaking subjects, like computer hackers, have something important to teach the authorities. Instead of regarding rule breakers as the enemy, they say, we ought to see them as potential allies in the effort to conduct ethical and scientifically sound clinical trials.

Supporters of the collaborative approach believe that "[m]otivation and commitment by subjects to fulfill their end of the bargain may hinge more on the appreciation of the research subject as a valued member of the research team than as a hired hand."[90] Thus the best way to proceed is to replace practices that devalue subjects' contributions with practices that demonstrate appreciation for what they do. And to learn what changes are needed, researchers need only consult the subjects themselves: "Who better than they to advise us on what makes for a 'rewarding' research experience?"[91]

In articles, interviews, and empirical studies, subjects have said a lot about what could be done to increase their commitment to trial requirements. Simple quality-of-life up-grades could go a long way toward improving the situation. Research facilities should be clean and comfortable. Subjects in on-site drug studies ought to have decent housing, good-quality food, and activities to lessen the boredom that some consider the worst part of the experience. Restrictions on their freedom should be limited to those required by study protocols or the demands of communal living. All subjects should receive free care and compensation for personal losses if they are injured in research.[92]

The research staff also has a major role in subjects' commitment to play by the rules. Subjects have high praise for studies conducted by personable and efficient teams.[93] Subjects are grateful when staff members pay attention and respond to their concerns. Subjects appreciate sincere ex-pressions of thanks for the pain, discomfort, and disruption they endure. Subjects value convenience too. In one survey of patient-subjects, staff flexibility in scheduling research visits was the number-one priority for a majority of the re-spondents.[94] Another study found that subjects were more cooperative and committed when staff members main-tained regular contact and supplied information on study progress.[95]

Another collaborative strategy is to adjust study re-quirements in ways that promote cooperation. Researchers adopted this strategy in the early years of the HIV/AIDS epidemic, when patients and activists rebelled against strict study rules. Activists eventually persuaded researchers and US Food and Drug Administration officials to become more flexible about trial methodology. For example, activists suc-cessfully challenged rigid trial eligibility criteria and strict rules governing subjects' medication use during trials.[96]

More recently, experts addressing nonadherence have urged researchers to consider strategies that make adherence easier, such as reducing study length and simplifying medication dosage rules.[97]

On a broader scale, the move to "adaptive" trial designs is a response to patients' reluctance to enroll in and complete studies that fail to offer them direct medical benefit. Besides the compliance problems I have described, researchers face a general shortage of patients willing to participate in clinical trials.[98] In an attempt to make trials more attractive to patients, researchers are developing study designs that allow randomization ratios, drug dosages, and other trial requirements to be adjusted during the trial based on accumulating trial data. These designs allow more subjects to be assigned to groups with superior outcomes.[99] Another relatively new approach is the "preference trial," which is designed to give at least some subjects an opportunity to choose which study intervention they will receive.[100] The reasoning is straightforward: "Subjects will simply find it easier to abide by the terms of protocols that pose less restrictive alternatives and require fewer personal sacrifices."[101]

Similar collaborative moves could promote adherence in phase 1 drug trials and other studies using healthy volunteers.[102] Is it really necessary, for example, to exclude vegetarians from phase 1 drug studies? Are other restrictive eligibility criteria applied more out of habit than genuine scientific need? Could some study tests, visits, dietary requirements, and other measures be eliminated without threatening the quality of the data? The research establishment should be open to changes that would make drug safety and other early-phase trials more subject-friendly while preserving study quality.

Community engagement is another collaborative development that could reduce rule-breaking. More researchers are asking prospective participants and their communities for advice on how to design and conduct trials. Community engagement can be used to explore how representatives of subject populations perceive risks, burdens, and other dimensions of proposed studies. By working with such representatives, research teams can "negotiate mutually acceptable practices with participants."[103] Subjects are more likely to cooperate with studies that take their needs and interests into account.[104] As one researcher commented, "participation that is actually enjoyable and interesting to research participants . . . has a higher likelihood of retaining them."[105]

STRENGTHENING SUBJECTS' COMMITMENT

Years ago, the philosopher Hans Jonas considered a fundamental moral question in human research: Under what conditions is it acceptable to put some individuals at risk for the benefit of others? According to Jonas, a human study is most acceptable when it involves subjects who fully identify with and understand the purpose of the research. Jonas argued that "the appeal for volunteers should seek this free and generous endorsement, the appropriation of the research purpose into the person's own scheme of ends."[106]

Rule-breaking subjects occupy a category distant from Jonas's ideal volunteer. No one, including members of the research community, should be shocked that many—perhaps most—subjects care more about their personal needs and circumstances than about the knowledge-seeking objectives of research. The question is what to do about rule-breaking. Big-brother monitoring may enable researchers to detect and deter misbehavior, but it is unlikely to increase subjects' personal commitment to the research mission. Vigorous guidance and instruction can also be effective, and in some cases will convince subjects to embrace research goals. But the most respectful way to strengthen their commitment is to minimize research practices that foster rule-breaking.[107]

Robert Helms founded *Guinea Pig Zero* "to rescue the value of the contribution that human subjects make to further biomedical research."[108] At times, even the most cynical and jaded professional guinea pigs express pride in the health advances they help bring about. Subjects may participate in trials for personal gain, but many are also altruistic.[109] In a hospitable and appreciative research environment, subjects may be more willing to put up with the requirements necessary to generate the good data that lead to medical progress.

Researchers seeking to reduce rule-breaking should listen to people like Robert Helms. They are the people who can describe both the origins of rule-breaking and the changes that would diminish this behavior. They are the people who can help researchers develop trials that are reasonable and humane. With subjects' help, researchers can develop a system that genuinely values study participants and strengthens their commitment to the research endeavor.

NOTES

1. Jeanne Marrazzo et al., "Tenofovir-Based Preexposure for HIV Infection among African Women," *New England Journal of Medicine* 372 (2015): 509–18.

2. Michael Saag, "Preventing HIV in Women—Still Trying to Find Their VOICE," *New England Journal of Medicine* 372 (2015): 564–65; Donald McNeil, "A Failed Trial in Africa Raises Questions About How to Test H.I.V. Drugs," *New York Times,* 5 February 2015. Retrieved February 19, 2015, from http://nyti.ms/1vtkZ1l.

3. Marrazzo et al., "Tenofovir-Based Preexposure," 516.

4. McNeil, "A Failed Trial." For more on subjects' perspectives on the trial, see Arlane van der Straten et al., "Perspectives on Use of Oral and Vaginal Antiretrovirals for HIV Prevention: The VOICE-C Qualitative Study in Johannesburg, South Africa," *Journal of the International AIDS Society* 17, supplement 2 (2014): 19146.

5. Kelly Servick, "'Nonadherence': A Bitter Pill for Drug Trials," *Science* 346 (2014): 288–89. Another investigator was quoted as saying, "It's very uncomfortable to grapple with this, because I think it challenges the very way we go about our business." Ibid., 288.

6. "Noncompliance" is another commonly used term for rule-breaking. Both terms are criticized on the grounds that they imply a hierarchical rather than egalitarian relation between the medical professional and layperson. John Steiner and Mark Earnest, "The Language of Medication-Taking," *Annals of Internal Medicine* 132, no. 11 (2000): 926–30; Soren Holm, "What Is Wrong with Compliance?," *Journal of Medical Ethics* 19 (1993): 108–10.

7. According to researcher Kenneth Schulz, requirements like randomization "annoy human nature." Some researchers try to control which subjects get assigned to specific study groups rather than leaving the assignment to chance. See Kenneth Schulz, "Subverting Randomization in Controlled Trials," *Journal of the American Medical Association* 274 (1995): 1456–58.

8. Sally Shumaker, Elizabeth Dugan, and Deborah Bowen, "Enhancing Adherence in Randomized Controlled Clinical Trials," *Controlled Clinical Trials* 21 (2000): 226S–32S, 226S.

9. Dorothy Smith, "Patient Nonadherence in Clinical Trials: Could There Be a Link to Postmarketing Patient Safety?," *Drug Information Journal* 46 (2012): 27–34, 28.

10. As one analyst told a reporter, "subjects are real people who act in their own interest, for money or to feel better"; they do not share the investigator's objective of generating "good, clean data." Servick, "'Nonadherence': A Bitter Pill," 289.

11. Rule violations have differing degrees of impact on research findings. But any violation of a rule designed to strengthen the validity of data presents a threat to study quality.

12. See David Wendler and Franklin Miller, "Deception in Clinical Research," in *The Oxford Textbook of Clinical Research Ethics*, ed. Ezekiel Emanuel et al. (New York: Oxford University Press, 2008), 315–24.

13. For evidence that deception by subjects is beginning to attract ethical attention, see David Resnik and David McCann, "Deception by Research Participants," *New England Journal of Medicine* 373 (2015): 1192–93.

14. Articles from the publication are collected in Robert Helms, ed., *Guinea Pig Zero: An Anthology of the Journal for Human Research Subjects* (New Orleans: Garrett County Press, 2002).

15. See Heather Edelblute and Jill Fisher, "Using 'Clinical Trial Diaries' to Track Patterns of Participation for Serial Healthy Volunteers in U.S. Phase I Studies," *Journal of Empirical Research on Human Research Ethics* 10, no. 1 (2015): 65–75; David McCann et al., "Medication Nonadherence, 'Professional Subjects,' and Apparent Placebo Responders: Overlapping Challenges for Medication Development," *Journal of Clinical Psychopharmacology* 35 (2015): 566–73.

16. Roberto Abadie, *The Professional Guinea Pig: Big Pharma and the Risky World of Human Subjects* (Durham, NC: Duke University Press, 2010).

17. David Resnik and Greg Koski, "A National Registry for Healthy Volunteers in Phase 1 Clinical Trials," *Journal of the American Medical Association* 305 (2011): 1236–37.

18. Abadie, *Professional Guinea Pig*, 81–82. See also McCann et al., "Medication Nonadherence"; Barbara Solow, "The Secret Lives of Guinea Pigs," *Independent Weekly*, February 9, 2000.

19. See Carl Tishler and Suzanne Bartholomae, "Repeat Participation among Normal Healthy Research Volunteers," *Perspectives in Biology and Medicine* 46 (2003): 508–20;

Glen Apseloff, Judy Swayne, and Nicholas Gerber, "Medical Histories May Be Unreliable in Screening Volunteers for Clinical Trials," *Clinical Pharmacology & Therapeutics* 60 (1996): 353–56; R. Hermann et al., "Adverse Events and Discomfort in Studies on Healthy Subjects: The Volunteer's Perspective," *European Journal of Clinical Pharmacology* 53 (1997): 207–14; Martin Patriquin, "Inside the Human Guinea Pig Capital of North America," *MacLean's* 122, no. 33 (2009); Solow, "Secret Lives"; Josh McHugh, "Drug Test Cowboys: The Secret World of Pharmaceutical Trial Subjects," *Wired*, April 24, 2007. Retrieved February 19, 2015, from http://www.wired.com/wired/archive/15.05/feat_drugtest.html. A University of Pennsylvania School of Medicine official admitted, "We ask subjects to disclose if they're participating in other trials—but if someone wants to lie, I won't necessarily know if they're simultaneously doing a trial across town." David Glenn, "Inside the Risky World of Drug-Trial 'Guinea Pigs,'" *Chronicle of Higher Education*, July 11, 2010.

20. Solow, "Secret Lives."

21. Abadie, *Professional Guinea Pig*, 60–61; Theresa Dulce, "Spanish Fly Guinea Pig: PPD Pharmaco, Where Slackers Refuel," in Helms, *Guinea Pig Zero*, 34–38, 34; Carl Elliott, "Guinea-Pigging," *New Yorker*, January 7, 2008; Solow, "Secret Lives."

22. Patriquin, "Inside"; Solow, "Secret Lives."

23. Patriquin, "Inside"; Apseloff, Swayne, and Gerber, "Medical Histories."

24. Abadie, *Professional Guinea Pig*, 60–61; Dulce, "Spanish Fly Guinea Pig," 37.

25. Hermann et al., "Adverse Events"; Laurie Cohen, "Stuck for Money: To Screen New Drugs for Safety, Lilly Pays Homeless Alcoholics," *Wall Street Journal*, November 14, 1996.

26. Abadie, *Professional Guinea Pig*, 24.

27. Jill Fisher, *Medical Research for Hire: The Political Economy of Pharmaceutical Clinical Trials* (New Brunswick, NJ: Rutgers University Press, 2009), 187; Roberto Abadie, "Tracking Professional Guinea Pigs," October 15, 2010. Retrieved February 19, 2015, from http://www.thehastingscenter.org/Bioethicsforum/Post.aspx?id=4933&blogid=140. For a

description of practices in studies offering payment to both healthy volunteers and patient-subjects, see Christine Grady et al., "An Analysis of U.S. Practices of Paying Research Participants," *Contemporary Clinical Trials* 26 (2005): 365–75.

28. Smith, "Patient Nonadherence," 30.

29. Michael Simmons et al., "Unpredictability of Deception in Compliance with Physician-Prescribed Bronchodilator Use in a Clinical Trial," *Chest* 118 (2000): 290–95.

30. Servick, "'Nonadherence': A Bitter Pill," 288. As the investigator in this study noted, even periodic blood tests cannot supply full information about subjects' adherence, because the tests capture a subject's status at just one point in time.

31. Fisher, *Medical Research for Hire*, 189.

32. Claire Bradley, "Designing Medical and Educational Intervention Studies," *Diabetes Care* 16 (1993): 509–18, 511. This researcher and a colleague commented, "despite having full information and giving consent, patients may still find themselves allocated to non-preferred treatments, which lowers their motivation to make the treatment work." C. Brewin and Claire Bradley, "Patient Preferences and Randomised Clinical Trials," *BMJ* 299 (1989): 313–15.

33. Anne Moyer, "Psychomethodology: The Psychology of Human Participation in Science," *Journal of Psychology of Science and Technology* 2 (2009): 59–72, 64.

34. Robert Finn, *Cancer Clinical Trials: Experimental Treatments & How They Can Help You* (Sebastopol, CA: O'Reilly, 1999), 18, 31. Subjects have a protected right to withdraw from research despite their earlier consent to participate. See "Federal Policy for the Protection of Human Subjects," 56 *Fed. Reg.* 28,016-17 (June 18, 1991). At the same time, individuals ought to enter trials with a good-faith intention to remain unless participation becomes too burdensome.

35. Steven Epstein, *Impure Science: AIDS, Activism, and the Politics of Knowledge* (Berkeley: University of California Press, 1996), 228. See also John Arras, "Noncompliance in AIDS Research," *Hastings Center Report* 20, no. 5 (1990): 24–32.

36. Moyer, "Psychomethodology," 64.

37. Ibid.

38. Smith, "Patient Nonadherence," 29.

39. Fisher, *Medical Research for Hire*, 192.

40. McHugh, "Drug Test Cowboys."

41. See Howard Mann, "Deception in the Single-Blind Run-In Phase of Clinical Trials," *IRB: Ethics & Human Research* 29, no. 2 (2007): 14–17; Franklin Miller, David Wendler, and Leora Swartzman, "Deception Research on the Placebo Effect," *PLoS Medicine* 2 (2005): e262.

42. Ginette Blackhart et al., "Assessing the Adequacy of Postexperimental Inquiries in Deception Research and the Factors that Promote Participant Honesty," *Behavior Research Methods* 44 (2012): 24–40; Marcella Boynton, David Portnoy, and Blair Johnson, "Exploring the Ethics and Psychological Impact of Deception in Psychological Research," *IRB: Ethics & Human Research* 35, no. 2 (2013): 7–13.

43. David Resnik and Elizabeth Ness, "Participants' Responsibilities in Clinical Research," *Journal of Medical Ethics* 38 (2012): 746–50.

44. Smith, "Patient Nonadherence."

45. A study of healthy volunteers showed that only about two-thirds promptly informed investigators about adverse events; the remainder withheld information temporarily or permanently. Hermann et al., "Adverse Events."

46. Epstein, *Impure Science*, 204. Subjects in the first placebo-controlled trial of AZT for HIV/AIDS admitted to sharing pills, but the trial still found that the drug was beneficial. Fortunately, AZT was so effective that subjects' sharing did not have a major impact on the study's outcome: "Noncompliance effectively blurred the differences between the treatment arm and the placebo arm, so the demonstration of a statistically significant difference became all the more impressive." Ibid., 238.

47. Mike Mitka, "FDA and Pharma Seek Better Ways to Assess Drug Safety, Efficacy in Clinical Trials," *Journal of the American Medical Association* 307 (2012): 2576–77, 2576. For specific cases in which initially approved dosages were later lowered due to safety concerns, see Smith, "Patient Nonadherence."

48. Apseloff et al., "Medical Histories," 356.

49. Eric Devine et al., "Concealment and Fabrication by Experienced Research Subjects," *Clinical Trials* 10 (2013): 935–48.
50. See Fisher, *Medical Research for Hire*, 182–83; Mitka, "FDA and Pharma," 2576.
51. See Servick, " 'Nonadherence': A Bitter Pill"; Stephen Rice and David Trafimow, "Known versus Unknown Threats to Internal Validity," *American Journal of Bioethics* 11, no. 4 (2011): 20–21.
52. Tishler and Bartholomae, "Repeat Participation."
53. Apseloff et al., "Medical Histories."
54. Ibid.
55. Abadie, *Professional Guinea Pig*, 74, 158; Adil Shamoo and David Resnik, "Strategies to Minimize Risks and Exploitation in Phase One Trials on Healthy Subjects," *American Journal of Bioethics* 6, no. 3 (2006): W1–13.
56. See Hermann et al., "Adverse Events."
57. Frank Miller and Alan Wertheimer, "Facing Up to Paternalism in Research Ethics," *Hastings Center Report* 37, no. 3 (2007): 24–34.
58. Kenneth De Ville, "The Case against Contract: Participant and Investigator Duty in Clinical Trials," *American Journal of Bioethics* 11, no. 4 (2011): 16–18, 17.
59. See Arras, "Noncompliance in AIDS Research."
60. Ibid., 25.
61. "The Cardinal Rules for Volunteering for Clinical Research," 2008. Retrieved February 19, 2015, from www.jalr.org/articles/rules.html. The website is a project of Paul Clough, a man who earns his living through clinical trial participation. See Alex O'Meara, *Chasing Medical Miracles: The Promise and Perils of Clinical Trials* (New York: Walker, 2009), 111–12.
62. G. Owen Schaefer, Ezekiel Emanuel, and Alan Wertheimer, "The Obligation to Participate in Research," *Journal of the American Medical Association* 302 (2009): 67–72, 68.
63. Robert Helms, "The What, Why, and How of the GPZ Grading System," in Helms, *Guinea Pig Zero*, 3–4. See also M. E. Hellard et al., "Methods Used to Maintain a High Level of Participant Involvement in a Clinical Trial," *Journal of Epidemiological and Community Health* 55 (2001): 348–51; "22 Nights and 23 Days: Diary of #1J, Drug Study Subject,"

2006. Retrieved February 19, 2015, from http://www.guin-eapigzero.com/23days.html. In a telling incident, after *Harper's Magazine* published some of Helms's report cards, a facility receiving a bad grade sued Helms for libel. See Abadie, *Professional Guinea Pig*, 52–53; Carl Elliott, "Research Volunteers Wanted. Earn Up to $7000," *Tin House*, Spring 2008, 103–106, 104.

64. Abadie, *Professional Guinea Pig*, 57, 139; Finn, *Cancer Clinical Trials*, 119; McHugh, "Drug Test Cowboys,"; Public Responsibility in Medicine & Research, "In Their Own Voices: A Discussion with Research Subjects Who Also Work in the Field of Subject Protections," 2010 Advancing Ethical Research Conference Proceedings. December 6–8, 2010, San Diego, California. Retrieved March 6, 2015, from https://www.conferencepassport.com/index.asp.

65. David Evans, Michael Smith, and Liz Willen, "Big Pharma's Shameful Secret," *Bloomberg Markets*, December 2005; Public Responsibility in Medicine and Research, "What Do Research Subjects Have to Say about Informed Consent?," National Harbor, Maryland, December 3, 2011. Retrieved April 26, 2013, from http://www.primr.org/ProgramArchives_Detail.aspx?id=2084.

66. Cambridge Clinical Trials, "Great Tips for Clinical Trials and Medical Trials Volunteer." Retrieved May 29, 2016, from http://www.cambridgeclinicaltrials.co.uk/great_tips.php. [the document is undated]

67. Abadie, *Professional Guinea Pig*, 10–11.

68. Elliott, "Research Volunteers Wanted," 104.

69. "22 Nights and 23 Days." In another sign of depersonaliza-tion, a volunteer reported that test-site staff called him by his trial number instead of his name. Abadie, *Professional Guinea Pig*, 29.

70. Abadie, *Professional Guinea Pig*, 157.

71. Fisher, *Medical Research for Hire*, 184–85.

72. Public Responsibility in Medicine and Research, "A Discussion with Research Subjects and Their Advocates," Nashville, Tennessee, November 15, 2009. Retrieved February 20, 2015, from http://www.meetingproceedings.com/2009/aerc/contents/index.asp.

73. Emily Elliot, "Panic at Penn," in Helms, *Guinea Pig Zero*, 29–33, 29.
74. Deborah Shelton, "Patients in Clinical Trials Don't Always Follow the Program," *American Medical News*, September 11, 2000.
75. Blackhart et al., "Assessing the Adequacy," 36.
76. Cynthia Rand and Mary Ann Sevick, "Ethics in Adherence Promotion and Monitoring," *Controlled Clinical Trials* 21, no. 5 (2000): 241S–47S, 245S.
77. Suz Redfearn, "Smart-Pill Technology Could Monitor Patient Compliance While Improving Clinical Trial Data Quality," April 4, 2011. Retrieved February 20, 2015, from http://www.centerwatch.com/news-online/2011/04/04/smart-pill-technology-could-monitor-patient-compliance-while-improving-clinical-trial-data-quality/.
78. Rand and Sevick, "Ethics in Adherence," 245S.
79. To be effective in our mobile society, registries need to cover wide geographic areas. See Resnik and Koski, "National Registry." For this reason, a private US venture called Verified Clinical Trials is attempting to establish a worldwide registry. "Verified Clinical Trials." Retrieved February 20, 2015, from http://www.verifiedclinicaltrials.com.
80. Shumaker, Dugan, and Bowen, "Enhancing Adherence," 228S.
81. Ibid.
82. Simmons et al., "Unpredictability of Deception," 294. See also Shumaker, Dugan, and Bowen, "Enhancing Adherence."
83. Sarah Edwards, "Assessing the Remedy: The Case for Contracts in Clinical Trials," *American Journal of Bioethics* 11, no. 4 (2011): 3–12, 3.
84. John Robertson, "Contractual Duties in Research, Surrogacy, and Stem Cell Donation," *American Journal of Bioethics* 11, no. 4 (2011): 13–14.
85. See Resnik and Ness, "Participants' Responsibilities," 748–49.
86. Smith, "Patient Nonadherence," 32.
87. Fisher, *Medical Research for Hire*, 193–98.
88. Shumaker, Dugan, and Bowen, "Enhancing Adherence," 229S.
89. Smith, "Patient Nonadherence," 30. Education won't always do the trick, however. Research coordinators told Jill Fisher that subjects who understand the scientific justification for

placebo-controlled trials aren't necessarily more accepting of assignment to a placebo group. Fisher, *Medical Research for Hire*, 189–90.

90. Nancy Reame, "Treating Research Subjects as Unskilled Wage Earners: A Risky Business," *American Journal of Bioethics* 1, no. 2 (2001): 53–54.

91. Ibid., 54.

92. Carl Elliott, "Justice for Injured Research Subjects," *New England Journal of Medicine* 367 (2012): 6–8; Rebecca Dresser, "Aligning Regulations and Ethics in Human Research," *Science* 337 (2012): 527–28.

93. See Helms, "La Crème de la Crème: Thomas Jefferson University," in Helms, *Guinea Pig Zero*, 8–9; Donno, "Awake with a Vengeance," in Helms, *Guinea Pig Zero*, 22–27. Roberto Abadie reports that in recent years, competition among re-search organizations has produced improved conditions in some locales but not others. He also reports that some guinea pigs don't like the "fancy sites" because they are too large and impersonal. Abadie, *Professional Guinea Pig*, 22–23. Subjects' comments on staff behavior bring to mind Dr. Michael Kahn's plea for more emphasis on basic etiquette in medical training: "The very notion of good manners may seem quaint or anachronistic, but it is at the heart of the mission of other service-related professions. The goals of a doctor differ in obviously important ways from those of a Nordstrom's em-ployee, but why shouldn't the clinical encounter similarly emphasize the provision of customer satisfaction through explicit actions?" Michael Kahn, "Etiquette-Based Medicine," *New England Journal of Medicine* 358 (2008): 1988–89, 1988.

94. Dan McDonald and Mary Jo Lamberti, "The Psychology of Clinical Trials: Understanding Physician Motivation and Patient Perception," *Centerwatch Research Brief*, October 4, 2006. Retrieved February 20, 2015, from http://www.centerwatch.com/news-online/article/566/the-psychology-of-clinical-trials-understanding-physician-motivation-and-patient-perception.

95. Hellard et al., "Methods Used to Maintain."

96. Epstein, *Impure Science*, 208–64; Rebecca Dresser, *When Science Offers Salvation: Patient Advocacy and Research Ethics* (New York: Oxford University Press, 2001), 21–43.

97. Servick, "'Nonadherence': A Bitter Pill," 289.
98. Neil Weisfeld, Rebecca English, and Anne Claiborne, *Envisioning a Transformed Clinical Trials Enterprise in the United States: Establishing an Agenda for 2020* (Washington, DC: National Academies Press, 2012).
99. William Meurer, Roger Lewis, and Donald Berry, "Adaptive Clinical Trials: A Partial Remedy for the Therapeutic Misconception?," *Journal of the American Medical Association* 307 (2012): 2377–78.
100. See Anna Floyd and Anne Moyer, "Effects of Participant Preferences in Unblinded Randomized Controlled Trials," *Journal of Empirical Research on Human Research Ethics* 5, no. 2 (2010): 81–93; Mary Janevic et al., "The Role of Choice in Health Education Intervention Trials: A Review and Case Study," *Social Science and Medicine* 56 (2003): 1581–94.
101. Arras, "Noncompliance in AIDS Research," 31. See also Finn, *Cancer Clinical Trials*, 117, describing a subject's success in convincing researchers to lower the number of biopsies in a trial.
102. Researchers addressing deception research note that there are "several ethical and methodological reasons why researchers should use deception sparingly." The inability to accurately detect subjects' awareness of deception is "yet another reason" for reducing use of this technique. Blackhart et al., "Assessing the Adequacy," 36.
103. Susan Cox and Michael McDonald, "Ethics Is for Human Subjects, Too: Participant Perspectives on Responsibility in Health Research," *Social Science and Medicine* 98 (2013): 224–31, 230.
104. John Lynch, "'Through a Glass Darkly': Researcher Ethnocentrism and the Demonization of Research Participants," *American Journal of Bioethics* 11, no. 4 (2011): 22–23; Vicki Marsh et al., "Beginning Community Engagement at a Busy Biomedical Research Programme: Experiences from the KEMRI CGMRC–Wellcome Trust Research Programme," *Social Science and Medicine* 67 (2008): 721–33.
105. Moyer, "Psychomethodology," 68.
106. Hans Jonas, "Philosophical Reflections on Experimenting with Human Subjects," *Daedalus* 98, no. 2 (1969): 219–47, 236.

107. Empirical evidence should be collected on the effectiveness of different strategies to reduce rule-breaking.

108. Abadie, *Professional Guinea Pig*, 51. In a panel presentation to researchers and IRB members and staff, Helms called on the audience to value what professional guinea pigs do for modern medicine: "Don't think about us as couch potatoes who just take money." Public Responsibility in Medicine and Research, "Discussion with Research Subjects."

109. Abadie, *Professional Guinea Pig*, 41; Leanne Stunkel and Christine Grady, "More than the Money: A Review of the Literature Examining Healthy Volunteer Motivations," *Contemporary Clinical Trials* 32 (2011): 342–52; Hermann et al., "Adverse Events."

5

Participants as Partners in Genetic Research

■□■

RESEARCH PROFESSIONALS HAVE traditionally controlled decisions about genetic research. But change is in the air. In this field, there is a move—often supported by researchers and ethicists—to look to research subjects and prospective subjects for ethical and policy guidance. Subjects, and the researchers and ethicists supporting them, envision a new model for genetic studies that is more compatible with the ideal of subjects and investigators as partners in research.

A variety of human studies fall under the heading of genetic research. This chapter focuses on research that involves the collection of DNA samples (also known as biospecimens) together with health information about the people providing the samples. Such samples and information are collected in research and also in medical settings, where blood, tissue, and other biological samples are taken in the course of delivering patient care. Samples and data from research subjects and patients are often stored in repositories known as

An earlier version of this chapter was published as "Public Preferences and the Challenge to Genetic Research Policy," in the *Journal of Law and the Biosciences* 1 (2014): 52–67.

biobanks. In many cases, stored samples and data are used in so-called secondary research projects investigating new scientific questions. Although it is possible to protect the identities of the individuals whose materials are used in genetic research, complete anonymity or security cannot be guaranteed.[1]

The move to empower subjects responds to a growing body of evidence about the views of genetic research subjects as well as of members of the public considering research participation. Information about these views comes from personal accounts, interviews, focus groups, surveys, and studies involving actual or prospective subjects. Both experienced and potential study participants have definite opinions on how they should be treated in genetic research.

Some researchers and ethicists contend that the data on subject and public preferences point to ethical deficiencies in existing research approaches. They also believe that failure to address subject and public preferences will decrease the number of individuals willing to participate in genetic research, thus jeopardizing its public health objectives.

People arguing for change say that current policy and practice fail to give due regard to the concerns and desires that many individuals who have joined or are considering joining genetic studies have about research uses of their biospecimens and associated health information.[2] Much of the discussion addresses three topics: (1) participants' control over research uses of their DNA samples and associated health information; (2) return of individual results to genetic research participants; and (3) compensation for participants in genetic research.[3] In this chapter, I describe evidence of actual and prospective subjects' views on these matters and arguments for moving toward a partnership model in genetic research.

Developments in genetic research could lead the way to changes in other types of human research that would enable subjects to exercise more control over the research process. At the same time, developments in genetic research reveal conflicts and ethical concerns that may arise in the move to a more genuine partnership model.[4]

SUPPORT FOR SUBJECT EMPOWERMENT

People contributing DNA samples and health information to genetic research, together with their researcher and ethicist allies, contend that certain accepted research practices fail to respect subjects. Subjects and their supporters propose new research approaches that would alter the status quo, giving genetic research participants a much greater role in determining how their data and samples are used.

I begin with one subject's personal account. Rebecca Fisher tells a stark and moving story about the gap between researcher and subject expectations. During the 1990s, Fisher and three of her relatives enrolled in a study that involved testing their DNA samples for a mutation of the *BRCA1* gene—a mutation that is associated with high rates of breast and ovarian cancer. Fisher had already had breast cancer, and the family wondered whether others were at risk. Fisher reported that during the three-year study period, "communication between the principal investigators and our family [was] practically nonexistent, and on those occasions when it did occur, it was almost exclusively at our behest. We received no regular status updates and, when we called or wrote to learn of any developments, our inquiries were met with annoyance, treated as an imposition—as though, once we relinquished our blood to these researchers, we were entitled to lay no further claim upon it."[5]

Fisher and her family felt used rather than respected in the research process. They had hoped to learn information relevant to their own health risks, but the researchers saw no reason to respond to their questions. While the researchers saw her family's blood and tissue samples as mere study materials, she and her relatives had a much different view. Although they joined the study to help others, they also assumed they would hear about the study's findings—findings that might have a bearing on their own health circumstances. But they "did not get anything back" from the researchers, except "the sense that we were part of a machine that might ultimately churn out some useful information for someone, somewhere." For this family, research participation produced "frustration and bitterness," as well as "a profound sense of betrayal."[6]

Another look at subject perspectives comes from interviews with a diverse group of people asked to contribute DNA samples and health information to research biobanks.[7] Fifty-seven people were interviewed; about half of them agreed to contribute to a biobank and half declined. Interviewers asked people about their understanding of biobank operations and their perceptions of biobank risks and potential benefits. But the interviewers also encouraged people to take the discussion in any direction they wanted. The unstructured discussion allowed ideas about ethical norms and concerns to emerge from the individuals who were considering whether to contribute to the biobanks rather than from the professionals conducting the interviews.

Several striking features became apparent in those discussions. Many of the prospective biobank contributors characterized their DNA "as a uniquely valuable source of information about themselves." They said they would share that information only if researchers agreed to certain terms, such as giving contributors opportunities to learn about data produced in studies of their biospecimens. Although people gave different opinions on whether they "owned" their DNA samples, many shared one person's view that the samples were "a piece of their essence."[8] The interviewers concluded that features like compensation and ongoing control over sample use will be required if biobanks are to attract the number of contributors needed for genetic studies. This led them to endorse a novel ethical and legal approach to biobank contributions, one built on the licensing of trade secrets.

I will go into the details of biobank contributor preferences later; here I simply want to call attention to this project's focus on research subject perspectives. According to the professionals who led the project, subjects should be more involved in decision-making about genetic research ethics. Experts have developed the existing ethical standards, they note, but they argue that this ought to change: "The rules, practices, and writings of medical and ethical experts embody and give voice to concerns that they think subjects have or, at least, ought to have. But there is little *a priori* reason to assume that the experts have it right, in the sense of giving accurate voice to their claimed constituency."[9] These professionals want their colleagues to stop thinking they can speak for subjects and instead let subjects speak for themselves. They believe "first, that people outside the community of sanctioned experts may have worthwhile ideas about how the practice of genetics should be carried out; and second, that those same people may prove to be competent partners in the enterprise."[10]

This group is not alone in calling for a more genuine research partnership. A growing number of researchers and ethicists are promoting arrangements in genetic research that give subjects more power over how research is conducted. For example, "participant-centric initiatives" use social media technologies to give genetic research subjects easy ways of locating and managing their personal research data. These initiatives replace the traditional one-time consent process with an interactive format that allows individual subjects to receive feedback on study outcomes and analysis, learn about new studies seeking enrollment, and communicate with researchers.[11]

Participant-centric initiatives put subjects at the center of decision-making about research. They reject the "black box" research model that so disturbed Rebecca Fisher's family, substituting for it "an ongoing active interaction between participants and researchers."[12] The initiatives demand "a substantial cultural shift in current research,"[13] a shift that "requires researchers to respect research participants as partners in the research rather than to see them as patients or passive providers of information and samples."[14]

Another new model further blurs the conventional boundaries between researchers and subjects. "Apomediated" research removes the investigator as research intermediary, adopting instead a peer exchange system in which subjects participate in data collection, interpretation, and other tasks traditionally assigned to research professionals.[15] The model relies on crowdsourcing through social media technologies and creates a framework that permits participants to organize their own research studies. For example, an online group called DIYGenomics led a study of the relationship between vitamin D and certain genetic mutations. Members of the group not only served as study subjects, they also designed the study, reported test results, compiled the data, and analyzed the findings.[16]

These emerging research models have been adopted in just a small number of studies to date. Many researchers see them as threats to the scientific enterprise.[17] And as I discuss later, studies conducted according to the new research models must still address ethical concerns about participants' privacy and their understanding of study information. At the same time, the new models are gaining public and professional attention, as well as support in some quarters. In 2015, an advisory group recommended participant-centric practices for a government-funded research initiative that would collect and store genetic and other health data from one million participants.[18] The new research models establish a general framework for empowering research subjects and for revising the specific research principles and practices I discuss below.

CONTROL OF BIOSPECIMENS AND ASSOCIATED DATA

Over the years, genetic researchers have at times studied biospecimens and health information without the informed consent or even awareness of the people whose materials were used. In some cases, materials that people agreed to contribute to one study have been used in different studies. In other cases, specimens and data collected from patients as part of their medical care have been used for research purposes.

These practices were accepted in the research community for decades, and ethicists and regulatory officials accepted them as well. A person's blanket consent to unspecified future research was seen as sufficient to authorize the use of their biospecimens and data in a variety of studies. Specimens and information collected in one research project could be used without consent in other studies if the sources' identities were not disclosed to the secondary researchers. Similarly, material obtained from patients in the course of medical care could be used in research without explicit permission as long as the patient's identity was protected. Experts thought that in these circumstances, people would have no reason to care about what was done with their DNA samples and data.

But there is increasing evidence that this expert judgment is wrong. Litigation over sample use supplies some of the evidence. Parents have filed lawsuits challenging the research use of blood samples collected as part of public health programs that screen newborns for genetic disease.[19] The Havasupai Indian tribe sued an Arizona State University researcher because blood samples that tribe members thought they were contributing to a genetic study of diabetes, a serious health problem in the Havasupai community, were also used in genetic studies on schizophrenia and the ancestry of tribe members.[20]

A broader picture of public attitudes comes from empirical work like the interview study I described earlier. Data from a variety of studies show that many people want to know what happens to material from and information about their bodies, and some have definite opinions on the types of research that should and should not be done with that material and information. Although some people are satisfied with the traditional approaches to genetic research, others are not.

Many studies have been conducted on public attitudes toward use of DNA samples in research; I will describe a few of them here. A large survey of members of the general public as well as focus groups drawn from the same population found majority support for requiring parents' informed permission to store blood samples obtained from newborns in health-related screening programs for future research use.[21] Another team conducting telephone interviews with 1,193 patients at academic medical centers found that 72 percent of the patients wanted to know about research uses of their leftover clinical samples (which are often referred to as "medical waste") even if the researchers would never learn the patients' identities.[22]

More information about public attitudes comes from a telephone survey involving 751 people living in the vicinity of a biobank being developed in Iowa. The biobank planned to collect biospecimens left over from medical tests and procedures; the specimens would be linked to patients' medical records, but data would be coded to protect patients' identities. Ninety percent of survey respondents said that some form of consent was required to store clinical samples and records. A majority also wanted some say about how their contributions would be used. Twenty-nine percent wanted the opportunity to consent to each specific study using their contribution, and another 25 percent wanted the chance to give "categorical consent," which allows individuals to decide which kinds of studies would be permissible. Forty-one percent preferred the option of giving one-time blanket consent to all research uses.[23]

A separate national survey conducted in 2007–8 examined public attitudes on research uses of biospecimens and health data. The survey team asked nearly five thousand people whether they would want the opportunity to decide about each specific research use of their contributions. Although 90 percent said they would be willing to contribute samples and data to a research biobank, nearly half wanted the power to decide about each specific use.[24]

Similarly, in focus groups with members of a Seattle-based healthcare delivery system, a research team found few people satisfied with the option of giving blanket consent to future research. Many focus group participants wanted the option of consenting to different categories of research, and nearly all thought that "researchers should seek study subjects' consent prior to implementing a substantive change in study procedures—for example, if data were to be used to study a different disease or if data were to be provided to a for-profit entity that had not been named in the original consent."[25]

Experienced genetic research subjects also want information about how their biospecimens and health information could be used in future research. In one survey, a University of Washington group asked 365 subjects in a genetic study about sharing deidentified data with other researchers. Eighty-six percent of the survey respondents were willing to have their data shared, but nearly all of them wanted an opportunity to decide the matter themselves. Ninety percent said that it was important for investigators to ask contributors for permission to share the data. Forty percent objected to an opt-out system that would allow data sharing unless a contributor affirmatively objected to sharing. Seventy percent objected to data sharing without notice or permission.[26] Although most agreed to the data sharing, many were concerned about whether their privacy would be sufficiently protected and whether the data would be used to advance the commercial interests of for-profit entities.[27]

Although quite supportive of the genetic research effort, most of these experienced research participants thought that people ought to be asked about wide data sharing. As the Washington group reported, "[b]eing given a choice about uses of their data that were not contemplated at the time of original consent was important . . . because the request represented a tangible demonstration of the researchers' trustworthiness and regard."[28]

Other empirical studies have produced similar findings.[29] Although some genetic research subjects and prospective subjects don't object to the traditional approaches, a sizable number do. Many people considering whether to contribute to genetic research want information about potential research uses of their biospecimens and data, as well as the authority to decide what uses are permissible. They want this information and authority when studies use their leftover medical samples and when their identities will be concealed from researchers. A significant number of people care about what happens to their biospecimens and to the genetic and health information associated with the specimens. These findings suggest that a successful genetic research effort may require changes in the conventional consent approaches governing research uses of biospecimens and associated health data.

RETURN OF GENETIC RESEARCH RESULTS

Like other forms of research, genetic research is conducted to advance knowledge. Although people enrolled in genetic studies sometimes receive personal benefits as a result of their participation, the studies' purpose is to produce information that could lead to improved care for future patients. Consistent with this purpose, the traditional recipients of study results have been scientists and physicians. In the past, researchers felt no obligation to give genetic study subjects information about either a study's overall results or the subjects' individual results.

By the 1990s, professionals' views about disclosure of overall study results were beginning to change. The change was partly a result of pressure from community and indigenous groups seeking greater control over research data produced in studies they were asked to join.[30] Although some researchers and ethicists took a paternalistic view, claiming that disclosure of study results might trigger unwarranted anxiety among subjects and lead them to seek unnecessary medical interventions, others came to believe that researchers had a responsibility to give interested subjects summaries of research results.[31] By 2009, an international survey of 343 genetic researchers found 90 percent agreeing that they had a duty to offer subjects information about overall research results.[32] Recognition of such a duty is consistent with the partnership model of human research, in which both researchers and subjects have a stake in learning the outcome of the study to which they have contributed.

The debate over returning individual research results is more divided, however. Many researchers and ethicists worry about psychological and other harms that could materialize if subjects learn about their individual results. Some oppose any return of individual results, and others want to return only "clinically actionable" results. Professionals generally see genetic research results as clinically actionable when "there are established therapeutic or preventive interventions or other available actions that have the potential to change the clinical course of the disease."[33] But empirical studies of potential research participants find that most think they should have an opportunity to learn a broader array of individual results.

The large 2007–8 US survey I described earlier asked people about their views on return of individual results in a proposed biobank project that would examine how genetic and other factors affect disease risk. Survey respondents said they would be most willing to join a project that returned individual results. The team conducting the survey reported that "[n]ine in ten respondents agreed that they would want to know their individual research results, and 91% wanted their individual research results about health risks 'even if there was nothing they could do about them.'"[34]

More details come from sixteen focus groups considering the same proposed biobank project. Members of the focus groups said they wanted accurate, valid, and actionable information about individual results, but many adopted a much broader concept of "actionable" than professionals tend to support. Not surprisingly, most focus group members wanted information relevant to potential medical treatment and disease prevention. But they expressed interest in receiving information relevant to other kinds of risks too, such as risks potentially applicable to their relatives and risks affecting reproductive decisions.

The focus group members also thought that information about currently untreatable and preventable conditions could be useful, given that future research advances could change the medical situation. Such information could help with financial planning and prompt them "to live life to its fullest now."[35] The information might lead them to enroll in studies of the relevant condition and become active in efforts to address environmental factors contributing to the condition. Comments like the following were common: "I'm volunteering some of my flesh for you to evaluate me. Tell me what's wrong with it. Not that you could do something about it necessarily, but at least let me know."[36]

People participating in another set of focus groups expressed similar views, offering many reasons for wanting results that fall short of the professional standard for clinical utility. Focus group members said that knowing about such results would empower contributors to genetic research, give them a sense of control, help their families, demonstrate researchers' respect for them, and lead them to feel more involved in the research. Some said the results "belong" to the biospecimen contributors, which makes it "unfair or wrong for researchers to know a person's [individual research results] without sharing them."[37] Many said they understood that the health significance of results is often uncertain and can change over time. But they "felt that the validity or reliability of the information was less important than researchers' transparency about their level of certainty about each result."[38] At the same time, although some focus group members expressed interest in receiving genetic information related to appearance and other nonmedical conditions, most called such results "frivolous."[39]

These surveys and focus groups tell us what members of the public believe they would consider in deciding whether to contribute samples and information for use in genetic research. Studies of actual research participants report similar findings. For example, a survey of people who had permitted samples to be stored for future research found that a substantial portion would want to know the results of a genetic study evaluating their risk of Alzheimer's disease, a condition that is largely untreatable at this time. One person commented, "the researcher would do us a disservice not to let us know, not to do so would be like the over-protective mother who doesn't let kids grow up."[40]

Rebecca Fisher, the breast cancer research subject I described earlier, also makes a compelling case for giving subjects the option of learning their individual results. Her contribution to research was motivated by altruism, yet she also expected something in return. Fisher wants researchers to develop "a more fulsome understanding of what . . . altruism means *to the giver*."[41] People who contribute to genetic research have "an entirely appropriate sense of entitlement" to learn what is discovered in the study, she declares, even if the results are of uncertain medical significance. Fisher makes this appeal to researchers: "Tell me what you know . . . even if you do not know what it means. Tell me because we are both human beings, and the new marketplace in which we suddenly find ourselves trades on the ultimate currency: our own cells."[42]

Misha Angrist, another genetic research participant, labels the return of results a "moral imperative." Angrist is both a research professional and a research subject. He has a PhD in genetics and a master's degree in genetic counseling. He was also an early contributor to the Personal Genome Project, a research project aimed at learning more about how genes and environment contribute to human traits.[43]

In an article on returning results, Angrist says it is "paternalistic and hypocritical" for researchers to refuse to return a broad range of results to interested participants.

Experts worried that participants will inflate the significance of genetic information have only themselves to blame, he contends, because the research community is largely responsible for the public's unrealistic perceptions of the implications of genetic findings. Moreover, he argues, worries about psychological harm, discrimination on the basis of genetics, and unnecessary medical procedures are based on assumptions rather than evidence.[44] Angrist believes that returning research results is a way to show respect for the autonomy of participants as well as to promote both their engagement in research and "a true abiding partnership between researcher and participant."[45]

Fisher, Angrist, and others voice strong opposition to unilateral professional control over the disclosure of research results. According to the empirical evidence, many of the people who have joined genetic studies or are prospective research contributors want to decide the matter for themselves. And their definition of useful information is broader than the definition most professionals support. As researcher Lynn Dressler observes, subjects who "consider themselves not just patients, but partners in research may consider return of results as a form of benefit-sharing or reciprocity not hinging on relevance to health."[46]

COMPENSATION FOR CONTRIBUTIONS

Money is at the heart of a third set of ethical issues relating to genetic research subjects. Should people contributing DNA samples and health information be paid? When their materials are used to develop a commercially valuable cell line or other product, should they receive a portion of the profits?

Traditionally, few contributors to genetic research received payment in any form, and courts have rejected research contributors' claims to a share of the profits from commercially lucrative research.

Many researchers and others argue that we should preserve and promote the existing system, which relies primarily on altruistic sample donation.[47] They recognize that it is acceptable, and sometimes necessary, to compensate patients and healthy volunteers for the time and effort it can take to provide samples and information for genetic research. But they oppose paying money for the samples and information themselves. Payment opponents say that assigning monetary value to genetic samples and information would dampen the altruism that often underlies the choice to contribute.

Opponents also stress practical difficulties in providing payment for samples and information. One payment option is to give all contributors a small amount when research materials are collected. The payment would have to be small at that point, because only a tiny number of contributions actually lead to revenue-generating products. A different option is to delay payment, reserving it for the rare cases in which research materials lead to valuable products. In this system, a few contributors would receive large payments, but the vast majority would receive nothing.

Many research professionals object to both payment options. Some say that small payments for all research materials "might not merely fail to incentivize patients, but might actually be scorned as an unfair or token reward."[48] And large payments to the lucky few whose materials were used to develop valuable products would also be problematic. Such an approach would not only be hard to administer, given the many years it can take to come up with a profit-making product; it would also be unjust to the many people who made similar research contributions but failed to hit the genetic product jackpot.[49]

Yet many potential research contributors are not worried about the negative effects of paying for genetic research materials. Certainly the concerns aren't shared by the individuals and patient groups who have claimed commercial interests in products developed from their DNA samples.[50] And empirical research reveals that many potential research contributors want to receive compensation for what they consider to be valuable materials, materials that are undeniably vital to the genetic research enterprise.

For example, compensation was a hot topic in the previously described interviews with fifty-seven people considering whether to contribute to genetic research biobanks. As a group, these interviewees "saw in their DNA something of unique value in the 'business' of medical research."[51] A number of them said that "easy money was their primary motivation" for agreeing to participate in a biobank offering $20 for a DNA sample.[52]

In the 2007–8 national survey I described earlier, researchers asked people how compensation would affect their willingness to contribute samples and information to a large biobank. Seventy-five percent said that monetary compensation was very or somewhat important to their choice whether to participate. Survey respondents were also asked about their responses to two possible payment amounts, $50 and $400. The higher compensation amount was a strong factor influencing willingness to participate.[53]

Other indications of contributor attitudes come from a Canadian project consulting members of the public about the "core values that should guide biobanking."[54] Participants spent four days learning about and discussing various issues, including payment to people contributing samples. Individuals proposed a variety of ways to compensate contributors, including fixed fees, a percentage of the proceeds from profitable research, and salaries for limited-term employment during the time samples are under study. The group eventually settled on a different arrangement: all tissue contributors should receive tax credits and relevant health information based on the research findings.

More information comes from a poll by the journal *Science* that asked readers whether researchers should be required to pay patients for tissue removed for therapeutic reasons in the course of their medical care. (This situation demands no extra time and effort of patients contributing the tissue.) Members of the research community are the primary readers of this journal, so it was surprising that 30 percent of the respondents thought that patients ought to be paid. One reader made the following comment: "When we recycle our trash at the curb, we receive a little kick-back on our trash costs. A decrement in our cost of medical services—certainly equal to the apportioned cost of tissue disposal—would psychologically have the same effect. We want a sense of control, courtesy, and justice, not an incalculable and probably unrealizable market value."[55]

In a letter to *Science* addressing the payment question, two economists disagreed with the prediction that payment would have a detrimental effect on altruism. The economists predicted that the "great majority of patients would likely be willing to donate waste tissue in exchange for either a fixed fee or a chance to share in the rewards of financially successful research."[56] They proposed that such arrangements would induce more individuals, both altruistic and nonaltruistic, to contribute. Purely altruistic contributors wouldn't necessarily be deterred, for they could donate their payments to a good cause.

Moreover, the economists observed, "blockbuster cell lines" produce great wealth for some researchers, while many others don't receive great financial rewards for their scientific work. If this sort of differential treatment is acceptable for researchers, the economists asked, why isn't differential treatment acceptable for DNA contributors too? And in what way would "such a system be less fair to patients than the current system, under which all revenues from tissue lines . . . accrue to the medical community?"[57]

So it appears that a significant number of people think that compensation for their DNA samples and associated information should be part of the genetic research system. Many subjects and potential subjects see their samples as essential to the research advances that improve healthcare and sometimes confer wealth on researchers and their employers. They don't necessarily expect to receive large payments, and altruism remains a major motivation for their research contributions. But they do want recognition that their contributions have value, and payment would constitute such recognition.

CHALLENGES TO THE PARTNERSHIP MODEL

Genetic research professionals developed traditional practices and policies with little input from research participants and the public. As a result, conventional approaches to consent, return of results, and payment fail to reflect the views of many actual and would-be research contributors. Thus far, many professionals have been reluctant to consider subjects' views in decision-making about genetic research. But this stance is becoming harder to defend.

Added costs and burdens for researchers are the major impediments to change. Measures giving people more control over research use of their materials, access to individual results, and compensation will be expensive and time-consuming. Contributor-centered policies will require research teams to establish communication systems that make it easy for subjects and researchers to interact. Tracking and distributing biospecimens according to contributors' research preferences will also present logistical challenges. Researchers will spend more time communicating with subjects than they have in the past, to discuss ongoing studies, new enrollment opportunities, and study results. Researchers providing individual results to study participants will need funds to cover high-quality genetic testing and professional time devoted to discussing results. Increased compensation to research contributors will also add to research budgets, and any effort to share profits with contributors might be difficult to implement.

Researchers may resent the added burdens, but what they see as costly and time-consuming frills are seen as basic necessities by many research contributors. For example, after some focus group participants learned that returning genetic research results would make the research more expensive, they replied that researchers should simply conduct smaller studies and use the savings to return results to contributors.[58] And reformers have proposed a variety of ways that genetic researchers can give more control to biospecimen contributors, offer them individual results, and compensate them without unduly compromising the research mission.[59]

It is also possible that at least some of the added research costs will be offset by savings in other areas. Based on the empirical data I have described, many people considering genetic research participation will react positively to the revised policies. As a result, recruiting research contributors could become easier and cheaper. And people who choose to contribute to research might feel more involved and appreciated in studies that offer them more control and compensation. This could in turn decrease dropout rates and increase participants' willingness to join future studies. Similarly, the opportunity to receive individual research results will give some participants an added incentive to complete study participation. Higher retention rates would allow studies to be completed faster and at lower cost.[60]

Several commentators think that that moving toward contributor-centered arrangements is in the genetic research community's self-interest. In proposing the return of at least some individual research results, law professor Hank Greely wrote: "Consider what happens after the first lawsuit by the bereaved family of a research subject whose life would have been saved had researchers revealed a risk they discovered. Whether or not the plaintiffs win, those researchers and their institutions will be branded as heartless, interested in subjects only as laboratory animals, and all biomedical research will feel the fallout."[61] Similarly, ethicist Tom Tomlinson predicts that public trust in and support of biobank research will increase if biobanks establish a system that gives contributors more information about and control over research uses of their materials.[62] Misha Angrist suggests that researchers will gain an advantage "in the marketplace for research participants" if they "proactively engage their participants, respond to their queries and make themselves available."[63]

Publicity about the Henrietta Lacks[64] case has heightened general awareness of research with DNA samples, and this awareness could affect the public's response to requests for genetic research subjects. Whether researchers like it or not, many people probably won't be willing to join studies unless they are given control of personal data, personally meaningful research results, and reasonable compensation for their contributions.

This is not to say that changes in genetic research practices would be completely beneficial for contributors. Some people might consent to wide sharing of their identifiable samples and information without understanding the potentially harmful consequences, such as privacy violations and barriers to obtaining life and disability insurance coverage.[65] Some could overestimate the benefits of genetic knowledge, and some could experience confusion or undue distress when they learn their research results.[66]

Effective education and counseling will be needed to address these problems. Measures to protect subjects from potential harm related to revised genetic research practices would be a defensible response to the expertise gaps, power differentials, and economic disparities that often characterize subject-researcher relationships. Moreover, the interests of the research community and the broader society must be taken into account in decisions about the best ways to respect subjects' preferences.

The task going forward is to determine where limits on complying with public and participant preferences are defensible, taking into account the views not only of research professionals but also of subjects and prospective subjects. What practices are justified by concern for subject protection? What level of donor control over biospecimens and associated data is reasonable? What concept of actionable results should guide the return of research results? What approaches would enable researchers to return research results in a meaningful yet affordable way?[67] What are fair and workable compensation arrangements?

As Rebecca Fisher reminds us, subjects are "fully one-half of the interaction" in genetics research.[68] For ethical and practical reasons, subjects and the public should have a greater role in determining how genetic research is conducted. Through becoming more inclusive, researchers, ethicists, and policymakers can develop defensible rules and practices that give due regard to the views of everyone whose contributions are essential to a successful genetic research endeavor.

NOTES

1. Laura Rodriguez et al., "The Complexities of Genomic Identifiability," *Science* 339 (2013): 275–76; Henry Greely, "The Uneasy Ethical and Legal Underpinnings of Large-Scale Genomic Biobanks," *Annual Review of Genomics and Human Genetics* 8 (2007): 343–64.
2. Existing US research regulations permit liberal research use of genetic samples and associated data without specific consent if the source's identity is protected. Gail Javitt, "Take Another Little Piece of My Heart: Regulating the Research Use of Human Biospecimens," *Journal of Law, Medicine & Ethics* 41 (2013): 424–39. The situation could change, however. In a 2015 Notice of Proposed Rulemaking, federal officials proposed revised regulations that would require at least

broad consent to research uses of samples and data whether or not the contributor could be identified. See Kathy Hudson and Francis Collins, "Bringing the Common Rule into the 21st Century," *New England Journal of Medicine* 373 (2015): 2293–96. A recently enacted federal law requires explicit parental informed consent to research uses of deidentified newborn blood samples. See Michelle Bayefsky, Katherine Saylor, and Benjamin Berkman, "Parental Consent for the Use of Residual Newborn Screening Bloodspots," *Journal of the American Medical Association* 314 (2015): 21–22. Existing regulations fail to include specific provisions on return of research results and on compensation and profits; as a result, researchers and institutional review boards currently have discretion over these matters. The 2015 Notice of Proposed Rulemaking includes a proposal to require researchers to disclose to prospective subjects whether research results, including individual results, will be provided, as well as the conditions under which results will be returned. Any plan to return research results would have to be submitted for IRB review. "Proposed Rules, Federal Policy for the Protection of Human Subjects," 80 *Fed. Reg.* 54, 053 (Sept. 8, 2015).

3. In August 2013, federal officials announced an agreement with the family of Henrietta Lacks, a woman whose biospecimen was used in research without her knowledge or consent. Lacks was a cancer patient in the early 1950s, but she made a long-standing research contribution. With the specimen, scientists developed a cell line that has been used by thousands of researchers worldwide. According to the 2013 agreement, any researcher seeking access to the cell line's genome sequence must first obtain permission from a committee that includes two Lacks family members. In reporting the agreement, officials wrote, "the relationship between researchers and participants is evolving: seeking permission emphasizes that participants are partners, not just 'subjects.'" The agreement did not award financial compensation to the Lacks family, however. Kathy Hudson and Francis Collins, "Family Matters," *Nature* 500 (2013): 141–42.

4. This chapter does not provide a comprehensive survey of empirical research on public and participant attitudes toward

the use of biospecimens, return of results, and compensation to contributors. Instead, it presents some of the findings suggesting that many (not all) actual and potential research subjects favor policies that differ from traditional genetic research policies.

5. Rebecca Fisher, "A Closer Look Revisited: Are We Subjects or Are We Donors?," *Genetics in Medicine* 14 (2012): 458–60, 458.

6. Ibid.

7. John Conley et al., "A Trade Secret Model for Genomic Biobanking," *Journal of Law, Medicine & Ethics* 40 (2012): 612–29.

8. Ibid., 619.

9. Ibid., 613.

10. Ibid., 615.

11. Jane Kaye et al., "From Patients to Partners: Participant-Centric Initiatives in Biomedical Research," *Nature Reviews/ Genetics* 13 (2012): 371–76.

12. Ibid., 373.

13. Ibid., 376.

14. Ibid., 375. Responding to research participants' desires for data control, Isaac Kohane and his colleagues developed a collaborative approach to genetic research they call the "Informed Cohort" (IC). People choose to enroll in the IC after an extensive disclosure and discussion process. Later, they give extra health information and biospecimens if they like, or withdraw from the cohort if they choose. They also decide whether their materials may be used in new studies. An oversight board communicates with IC participants; this board is multidisciplinary and includes research participants. According to Kohane's group, the approach treats "patients as partners in research rather than passive, disenfranchised purveyors of biomaterials and data." Isaac Kohane et al., "Reestablishing the Researcher-Patient Compact," *Science* 316 (2007): 836–37, 837. For a description of a program that has adopted elements of this approach, see Courtney Kronenthal, Susan Delaney, and Michael Christman, "Broadening Research Consent in the Era of Genome-Informed Medicine," *Genetics in Medicine* 14 (2012): 432–46.

15. Dan O'Connor, "The Apomediated World: Regulating Research When Social Media Has Changed Research," *Journal of Law, Medicine & Ethics* 41 (2013): 470–83. See also Valerie Gutmann Koch, "PGT and Me: Social Networking-Based Genetic Testing and the Evolving Research Model," *Health Matrix* 22 (2012): 33–74.

16. See O'Connnor, "Apomediated World," 471, 473.

17. Sharon Terry and Patrick Terry, "Power to the People: Participant Ownership of Clinical Trial Data," *Science Translational Medicine* 3 (2011): 1–4.

18. Dixie Baker et al., "Participant Engagement, Data Privacy, and Novel Ways of Returning Information to Participants," NIH Workshop on Building a Precision Medicine Research Cohort, Bethesda, MD, February 11–12, 2015. Retrieved March 13, 2015, from http://www.nih.gov/precisionmedicine/workshop.htm. The advisers favored participant control over data and sample use, as well as return of individual research results to participants. The cohort project is described in Francis Collins and Harold Varmus, "A New Initiative on Precision Medicine," *New England Journal of Medicine* 373 (2015): 793–95; Jocelyn Kaiser, "NIH Plots Million-Person Megastudy," *Science* 347 (2015): 817.

19. See Javitt, "Take Another," 431.

20. See Michelle Mello and Leslie Wolf, "The Havasupai Indian Tribe Case—Lessons for Research Involving Stored Samples," *New England Journal of Medicine* 363 (2010): 204–7. Rebecca Skloot, author of the best-selling book, *The Immortal Life of Henrietta Lacks*, said that during her book tours, "people ask at every stop ... how they can find out what is being done with the blood or biopsy they may have left at a hospital." She told a journalist that people have "this sense of, 'it's a piece of my body, and I want to know what's happening to it.'" Amy Harmon, "Where'd You Go with My DNA?," *New York Times*, April 24, 2010. Retrieved March 15, 2015, from http://www.nytimes.com/2010/04/25/weekinreview/25harmon.html.

21. Jeffrey Botkin et al., "Public Attitudes Regarding the Use of Residual Newborn Screening Specimens for Research," *Pediatrics* 129 (2012): 231–38.

22. Sara Chandros Hull et al., "Patients' Views on Identifiability of Samples and Informed Consent for Genetic Research," *American Journal of Bioethics* 8, no. 10 (2008): 62–70.

23. Christian Simon et al., "Active Choice but Not Too Active: Public Perspectives on Biobank Consent Models," *Genetics in Medicine* 13 (2011): 821–31. Some prospective and actual subjects who support the blanket-consent model may not realize what blanket consent can cover. When a survey team asked a representative sample of the US population about consent to biobank donation, 68 percent of the people responding said they would be willing to give blanket consent to donation. But that figure declined after people learned that certain kinds of morally controversial studies may involve the use of biospecimens, such as research related to abortion methods, commercial drug development, and genetic predispositions to violence. These findings suggest that some people who say they favor blanket consent do not understand the different ways that their samples and data might be used in research. Tom Tomlinson et al., "Moral Concerns and the Willingness to Donate to a Research Biobank," *Journal of the American Medical Association* 313 (2015): 417–18.

24. Juli Murphy et al., "Public Perspectives on Informed Consent in Biobanking," *American Journal of Public Health* 99 (2009): 2128–34.

25. Susan Trinidad et al., "Informed Consent in Genome-Scale Research: What Do Prospective Participants Think?," *AJOB Primary Research* 3, no. 3 (2012): 3–11.

26. Susan Trinidad et al., "Research Practice and Participant Preferences: The Growing Gulf," *Science* 331 (2011): 287–88.

27. Evette Ludman et al., "Glad You Asked: Participants' Opinions of Re-consent for DbGaP Submission," *Journal of Empirical Research on Human Research Ethics* 5, no. 3 (2010): 9–16.

28. Trinidad et al., "Research Practice," 288.

29. See B. A. Tarini et al., "Not without My Permission: Parents' Willingness to Permit Use of Newborn Screening Samples for Research," *Public Health Genomics* 13 (2010): 125–30; Kieran O'Doherty, Alice Hawkins, and Michael Burgess, "Involving Citizens in the Ethics of Biobank Research: Informing

Institutional Policy through Structured Public Deliberation," *Social Science and Medicine* 75 (2012): 1604–11.

30. Rebecca Dresser, *When Science Offers Salvation: Patient Advocacy and Research Ethics* (New York: Oxford University Press, 2001), 22–43.

31. Ann Partridge and Eric Winer, "Informing Clinical Trial Participants about Study Results," *Journal of the American Medical Association* 288 (2002): 363–65.

32. Fiona Miller et al., "What Does 'Respect for Persons' Require? Attitudes and Reported Practices of Genetics Researchers in Informing Research Participants about Research," *Journal of Medical Ethics* 38 (2012): 48–52. Despite widespread acknowledgment of a duty to return overall study results, "return of aggregate results is still an uncommon practice in the United States." Lynn Dressler, "Disclosure of Research Results from Cancer Genomic Studies: State of the Science," *Clinical Cancer Research* 15 (2009): 4270–76.

33. Richard Fabsitz et al., "Ethical and Practical Guidelines for Reporting Genetic Research Results to Study Participants," *Circulation: Cardiovascular Genetics* 3 (2010): 574–80. Another group took a similar position on return of results in studies using biobank contributions. Susan Wolf et al., "Managing Incidental Findings and Research Results in Genomic Research Involving Biobanks and Archived Data Sets," *Genetics in Medicine* 14 (2012): 361–84.

34. David Kaufman et al., "Subjects Matter: A Survey of Public Opinions about a Large Genetic Cohort Study," *Genetics in Medicine* 10 (2008): 831–39, 835.

35. Juli Murphy et al., "Public Expectations for Return of Results from Large-Cohort Genetic Research," *American Journal of Bioethics* 8, no. 11 (2008): 36–43, 40.

36. Ibid., 40.

37. Juli Murphy Bollinger et al., "Public Preferences Regarding the Return of Individual Genetic Research Results," *Genetics in Medicine* 14 (2012): 451–57, 456.

38. Ibid., 456.

39. Ibid., 454–55.

40. David Wendler and Rebecca Pentz, "How Does the Collection of Genetic Test Results Affect Research Participants?,"

American Journal of Medicine Genetics Part A 143 (2007): 1733–38, 1736. See also David Shalowitz and Franklin Miller, "Communicating the Results of Clinical Research to Participants: Attitudes, Practices, and Future Directions," *PLoS Medicine* 5 (2008): 714–20.

41. Rebecca Fisher, "A Closer Look: Are We Subjects or Are We Donors?," *American Journal of Bioethics* 8, no. 11 (2008): 49–50.

42. Ibid., 49.

43. The project is described at www.personalgenomes.org. Angrist wrote a book about the project and his experience as a participant. Misha Angrist, *Here Is a Human Being: At the Dawn of Personal Genomics* (New York: Harper Perennial, 2011).

44. Because the practice of returning individual research results is relatively new, few teams have evaluated the effects of disclosure on subjects. One group that performed such an evaluation reported that subjects were highly satisfied with the disclosure process and reported no significant psychological harm three months after they learned their results. Kurt Christensen et al., "Disclosing Individual CDKN2A Research Results to Melanoma Survivors: Interest, Impact, and Demand on Researchers," *Cancer Epidemiology, Biomarkers & Prevention* 20 (2011): 522–29.

45. Misha Angrist, "You Never Call, You Never Write: Why the Return of 'Omic' Results to Research Participants Is Both a Good Idea and a Moral Imperative," *Personalized Medicine* 8 (2011): 651–57.

46. Dressler, "Disclosure of Research Results," 4275.

47. For example, Robert Truog, Aaron Kesselheim, and Steven Joffe, "Paying Patients for Their Tissue: The Legacy of Henrietta Lacks," *Science* 337 (2012): 37–38.

48. Ibid., 38.

49. Ibid.

50. Jon Merz et al., "Protecting Subjects' Interests in Genetics Research," *American Journal of Human Genetics* 70 (2002): 965–71.

51. Conley et al., "Trade Secret Model," 622.

52. Ibid., 620.

53. Kaufman et al., "Subjects Matter," 835, 838.

54. Heather L. Walmsley, "Stock Options, Tax Credits, or Employment Contracts Please! The Value of Deliberative Public Disagreement about Human Tissue Donation," *Social Science & Medicine* 73 (2011): 209–16.

55. Heidi Draffin, "Readers' Poll Results: Paying for Tissue," *Science* 338 (2012): 328.

56. Scott Kominers and Gary Becker, "Paying for Tissue: Net Benefits," *Science* 337 (2012): 1292.

57. Ibid. See also John C. Bear, "'What's My DNA Worth, Anyway?' A Response to the Commercialization of Individuals' DNA Information," *Perspectives in Biology and Medicine* 47 (2004): 273–89.

58. Bollinger et al., "Public Preferences."

59. See Kaye et al., "From Patients to Partners"; Kohane et al., "Reestablishing"; Greely, "Uneasy Ethical and Legal"; J. Scott Roberts et al., "Returning Individual Research Results: Development of a Cancer Genetics Education and Risk Communication Protocol," *Journal of Empirical Research on Human Research Ethics* 5, no. 3 (2010): 17–30; Merz et al., "Protecting Subjects' Interests"; Bear, "'What's My DNA Worth.'" Two experts argue that the debate over return of results "should be widened to a discussion about the availability of funding to create the infrastructure for a communication system regarding the disclosure of whole genome sequencing and whole exome sequencing findings to research participants." Felicitas Holzer and Ignacia Mastroleo, "Support for Full Disclosure Up Front," *Hastings Center Report* 45, no. 1 (2015): 3.

60. See Kaufman et al., "Subjects Matter," 35; Ludman et al., "Glad You Asked"; Christensen et al., "Disclosing."

61. Greely, "Uneasy Ethical and Legal," 360.

62. Tom Tomlinson, "Respecting Donors to Biobanks," *Hastings Center Report* 43, no. 1 (2013): 41–47.

63. Angrist, "You Never Call," 652.

64. See note 3.

65. See O'Connor, "Apomediated World"; Misha Angrist, "Eyes Wide Open: The Personal Genome Project, Citizen Science and Veracity in Informed Consent," *Personalized Medicine* 6 (2009): 691–99.

66. See Ellen Wright Clayton and Lainie Friedman Ross, "Implications of Disclosing Individual Research Results of Clinical Research," *Journal of the American Medical Association* 295 (2006): 37.
67. One group reported that a program for disclosing research results that received high satisfaction rates from participants "required more than 2 hours and 30 minutes and more than $1,300 per completed disclosure to execute." Christensen et al., "Disclosing," 527.
68. Fisher, "Closer Look Revisited," 459.

6

Terminally Ill Patients and the "Right to Try" Experimental Drugs

■□■

IN 2014, state legislatures were asked to recognize a new legal right for terminally ill patients—a right to try experimental drugs. Because these drugs have not been fully evaluated in human studies, it is unclear whether they are safe and effective. Yet some patients still want to try them, arguing that they have no other good options left. Right-to-try advocates wanted states to help these patients by making it easier to get the unproven drugs. Many lawmakers were persuaded, and by the end of 2015, nearly half the states had passed right-to-try laws.[1]

Right-to-try laws are the latest development in a decades-long struggle between advocates of liberal access to experimental drugs and defenders of access restrictions. According to liberal-access advocates, terminally ill

An earlier version of this chapter was published as "The 'Right to Try' Investigational Drugs: Science and Stories in the Access Debate," *Texas Law Review* 93 (2015): 1631–57.

patients shouldn't have to enroll in research to gain access to experimental drugs.

But right-to-try opponents say the laws will do more harm than good, exposing vulnerable patients to risky and ineffective measures. Opponents also argue that right-to-try laws pose an unacceptable threat to the larger group of patients who benefit from receiving drugs that have been thoroughly tested. They predict that if terminally ill patients can easily obtain experimental drugs without enrolling in research, fewer patients will choose to participate in the studies that show which drugs actually help people live longer and better lives.

Scientists and policy analysts criticizing right-to-try laws cite data on the risks and low success rates of experimental drugs as well as the need for a rigorous drug evaluation system. But in the access debate, data and abstract policy considerations go only so far. Liberal-access advocates use a different strategy, one that highlights patients' stories.

To support their cause, right-to-try advocates tell heart-rending stories about terminally ill patients seeking experimental drugs and about patients who died after failing to obtain such drugs. Advocates know that patients' stories "have the power to reach a public who has little understanding of the research enterprise."[2] The access debate shows how persuasive patients' experiences can be in shaping legislative and public opinion about a research ethics issue.

The problem with the right-to-try advocates' strategy is that their examples are one-sided. Advocates don't talk about the patients who do badly after trying experimental treatments. They don't talk about the patients who suffer when the drug approval process is extended because drug studies can't enroll enough subjects. Stories illustrating the harm that can come from liberal access belong in the debate too. The debate over right to try should include examples of patients who pay a high price for liberal access to experimental measures.

In this chapter, I examine the right-to-try controversy and the role patients' experiences play in the controversy. First I review the history of regulation of experimental drugs and the current rules governing access to such drugs. Then I present the ethical and policy arguments for and against liberal access rules.

To illustrate the potential benefits and harms of trying experimental measures, I tell a variety of patients' stories. I also consider interview and survey data examining patients' attitudes toward and experiences with experimental interventions. My goal is to present a balanced picture of what can happen when terminally ill patients try experimental drugs. Information like this is essential to developing access policies that truly promote patients' interests.

HOW THE GOVERNMENT REGULATES EXPERIMENTAL DRUGS

Drug Evaluation

Federal law prohibits companies from marketing new drugs without approval from the Food and Drug Administration (FDA). To obtain FDA approval, companies must first submit evidence that drugs are both safe and effective for medical use.[3]

Evidence from human studies is necessary to demonstrate drug safety and effectiveness. Before a company may conduct those studies, the FDA must issue an exemption allowing the company to test the experimental drug. Officials at the FDA review study proposals to make sure that they are based on adequate scientific evidence and will not expose research subjects to unacceptable risk.

The FDA divides drug studies into three phases. Phase 1 trials are typically conducted on twenty to eighty human subjects. These trials supply initial information about a drug's adverse effects in humans and help researchers determine a reasonably safe drug dosage. Although phase 1 trials are not designed to evaluate a drug's potential benefit, they sometimes produce preliminary evidence about this.

If a drug appears to have an acceptable safety profile, the FDA will permit a phase 2 study. Up to several hundred subjects with the disease that the drug is targeting participate in phase 2 trials. In these trials, researchers continue to collect information on side effects and risks, but they also look for evidence of the drug's effectiveness. If phase 2 evidence suggests that the drug presents an acceptable balance of risks and potential benefits, officials allow the company to go forward with phase 3 trials, which evaluate safety and effectiveness in a larger number of patients. If phase 3 trials have acceptable results, the company can then seek FDA approval to market the drug.[4]

About 70 percent of the drugs that go through phase 1 testing are found safe enough to advance to phase 2 trials. But many of those drugs fail to demonstrate enough promise to advance to phase 3 testing. Only about one-third of drugs are successful in both phase 1 and 2 trials,[5] and as one expert put it, the "bottleneck" is in phase 2.[6]

Not many drugs make it to final approval. In 2013, an expert group estimated that about one in six drugs that enter human testing is approved for medical use.[7] A 2014 study was even less encouraging, putting the figure at one in ten.

Cancer drugs, which are often the focus of patient access requests, have a lower-than-average success rate. The 2014 study found that one in fifteen experimental cancer drugs tested in humans was eventually approved by the FDA.[8] And even FDA-approved cancer drugs fail to help many patients.[9]

History of FDA Access Policy

Not all terminally ill patients are eligible to participate in drug trials. Because companies test drugs for a limited number of medical uses, patients must meet specific eligibility criteria to enter a trial. Excluded from trials are patients whose illness differs from the disease the drug is targeting. A patient's age, physical condition, or exposure to previous treatments can lead to trial ineligibility too. Some patients live too far away from trial centers to participate.

Not every patient who is eligible to participate in trials chooses to enroll. Some are unwilling to accept extra hospital visits, tests, and other study requirements. And as I described in chapter 3, patients at times refuse to participate because they fear they will be assigned to a control group that will receive an inactive placebo or a standard therapy with low success rates.[10]

Patients who are unable or unwilling to enroll in clinical trials may still want to try investigational drugs. In what are popularly known as "compassionate use" programs, the FDA permits certain patients to try such drugs without enrolling in studies.

The HIV/AIDS epidemic gave rise to the first broad compassionate-use program. In 1987, the FDA issued regulations giving drug access to patients with any serious or immediately life-threatening condition. To qualify, patients had to have no other reasonable options, including the option of enrolling in a drug study. Doctors and drug companies could apply for FDA permission to give an experimental drug to a qualified patient.

Under the 1987 regulations, FDA officials ordinarily permitted patients to try drugs during or following completion of phase 3 trials. But in "appropriate circumstances," including the presence of an immediately life-threatening condition, drugs could be made available during phase 2 testing. The regulations said a patient's request could be denied if the existing scientific evidence failed to provide a reasonable basis for concluding that the drug could be effective or if the drug presented "an unreasonable and significant additional risk of illness or injury."[11]

The compassionate-access regulations also required documentation of patients' informed consent. An institutional review board (IRB) had to approve patients' requests as well. In emergency situations, the FDA could permit compassionate use on a temporary basis without a formal request. The regulations allowed companies to recover the direct costs of supplying patients with drugs, but did not allow the companies to profit from the transaction.

Although hundreds of patients received experimental drugs through the FDA program, critics complained that it was applied unfairly and inconsistently. They also said that the process was so demanding and time-consuming that many terminally ill patients were unable to benefit from it.

A patient advocacy organization called the Abigail Alliance for Better Access to Developmental Drugs eventually challenged the FDA regulations. The alliance was founded by the father of Abigail Burroughs, a young woman who tried to obtain two experimental drugs for cancer treatment.[12]

Burroughs wasn't eligible to participate in trials that were evaluating the drugs, and the companies refused to include her in their limited compassionate-use programs.[13] Although the FDA wasn't responsible for her inability to get the drugs, the alliance argued that the FDA's refusal to allow companies to profit from selling unapproved drugs was keeping companies from meeting patients' compassionate-use requests.

The alliance turned to the federal courts for relief. It filed a complaint asserting that the FDA's compassionate-access rules violated the terminally ill patient's constitutionally protected right to obtain drugs that have completed phase 1 testing. The case took several twists and turns, but the courts ultimately rejected this constitutional claim.[14]

In a separate development, however, the FDA revised its regulations in 2009. Most of the requirements in the new rules resemble the 1987 rules, but there are a few notable changes.[15] The most significant changes allow patients to obtain drugs earlier in the testing process. In most cases, FDA officials will make drugs available to patients with an "immediately life-threatening disease" during phase 2 trials. In certain cases, however, officials may make drugs available before phase 1 testing is complete. And in exceptional circumstances, officials may make a drug available to patients in the absence of any data on its human effects.[16] Thus the 2009 FDA policy is in some ways more liberal than the Abigail Alliance's proposal to permit compassionate use after phase 1 testing.

State Right-to-Try Laws

Despite its liberal provisions, the current FDA policy fails to satisfy some patients and advocates. In 2014, the Goldwater Institute, a nonprofit organization, developed a model bill "to protect the fundamental right of people to try to save their own lives."[17] Most state right-to-try laws are based on this model bill.[18]

State right-to-try laws vary, but they all seek to give terminally ill patients compassionate access to experimental drugs without the FDA's permission. The laws permit companies to provide drugs that have completed phase 1 testing to patients whose physicians have recommended the drugs. Patients must give written informed consent to drug use, and companies may charge patients for the costs of supplying the drugs.

All state right-to-try laws bar state licensing boards from taking disciplinary action against physicians who comply with the laws' requirements. Some right-to-try laws give added legal protection to medical professionals and drug companies that provide drugs to patients. But these laws do not require companies to supply drugs to patients, nor do they require patients' health insurance companies to cover the costs of obtaining the drugs.[19]

THE POLICY DEBATE

The people behind right-to-try laws want to do away with FDA review of compassionate-use requests. They argue that patients and doctors can make good decisions on their own and that FDA review requirements are too paternalistic. But people defending access restrictions have a different view. They argue that both patients and the public benefit from FDA oversight. They also see right-to-try laws as "nothing but feel-good placebos" that will have no real impact on patients' lives.[20]

Individual Autonomy versus Patient Protection

According to right-to-try advocates, access to experimental drugs is not a scientific or public health concern but a matter for patients and their doctors to decide. Once a drug has undergone phase 1 testing, access advocates believe that doctors are competent to determine whether it is promising enough for patients to try.[21] Advocates reject claims that patients need FDA protection because they are desperate and vulnerable, arguing that such claims demean people who are fully capable of making their own treatment decisions. To access advocates, "no-one is better placed than the person with the condition, or their family, to make a judgment about the level of risk that is worthwhile."[22]

Right-to-try advocates criticize the FDA's substantive limits on compassionate use, but what they really object to is the review requirement itself. Officials at the FDA grant nearly every patient's request for compassionate access and do so quickly in urgent cases.[23] But preparing a request can be time-consuming. Right-to-try advocates say that the burden of preparing a request keeps overworked doctors and drug company officials from seeking compassionate access. They also say that the IRB review requirement is an undue obstacle to compassionate access.

According to right-to-try advocates, many patients who could benefit from trying experimental drugs are deprived of help because the FDA insists on being involved in the decision. As one advocate complained, "FDA's long, costly, and burdensome process makes it difficult for patients to get the medications that may save their lives."[24]

Right-to-try opponents paint a very different picture. They point to data showing that many terminally ill patients don't understand the risks of trying experimental drugs. According to the data, patients commonly overestimate the odds that such drugs will lengthen or improve their lives. Indeed, one medical expert says that the entire right-to-try campaign relies on a mistaken conception of experimental drugs as "miracle" treatments.[25]

Opponents also say the right-to-try campaign ignores the suffering that can come from trying experimental drugs. They don't believe compassionate access is truly compassionate. To the advocates who ask, "What's the harm?" in granting patients a right to try, one expert responded, "If there's anything worse than dying of a terminal illness, it's dying of a terminal illness and suffering unnecessary complications or pain for no benefit and having to pay for the medications causing the complications yourself."[26]

Right-to-try opponents see terminally ill patients as vulnerable people who need more, not less, protection. Some want rules requiring closer monitoring for patients receiving experimental measures and clear criteria for stopping those measures. As one right-to-try opponent put it, instead of adopting rules that expose more terminally ill patients to harm and disappointment, "the gate to access experimental treatments must be closed enough to prevent medical interventions that impose excessive harm."[27]

Individual versus Societal Interests

Besides disagreeing on the proper balance of patient freedom and protection, right-to-try advocates and opponents disagree on the proper balance of individual and societal interests. Opponents insist that a rigorous clinical trial system is essential to determining whether drugs are safe and effective enough to be approved for general patient use. Making drugs easily available outside research could threaten that system. Because relatively few patients enroll in studies, it often takes many years to determine the quality of experimental drugs. If more patients can obtain drugs outside research, there will be even fewer willing to sign up for the studies that show which drugs can actually help patients.[28]

Under existing FDA regulations, officials may approve compassionate use only if it "will not interfere with the initiation, conduct, or completion of clinical investigations that could support marketing approval" of the experimental drug.[29] Right-to-try advocates say that excluding study-eligible patients is an unethical sacrifice of their interests to promote the greater good. According to the advocates, a rule that "forces people to go into clinical trials if they want access to the only possibly lifesaving drugs" is unacceptably coercive.[30]

Right-to-try opponents see the situation quite differently. They argue that the terminally ill patient's interest in trying experimental drugs is less important than the public's interest in maintaining a high-quality drug review system. Because liberal access will make it harder to conduct clinical trials, the drug review process will be extended. Widespread patient access will be delayed, and many more patients will suffer, because it will take longer to get drugs fully approved.[31]

Public health experts defending access limits believe that "the public, as a body, merits protection from interference by individual members of society."[32] One characterized the Abigail Alliance's access position as an "aggressively individualistic view, one that breathtakingly slights the public's interest in drug safety."[33] Right-to-try opponents say the FDA's current compassionate-access rules allow many patients to try experimental drugs, striking a reasonable balance between individual and public health needs.[34]

Doubts about Impact

According to right-to-try advocates, eliminating FDA oversight will greatly increase patients' access to experimental drugs, giving them real opportunities to save their lives. As one right-to-try advocate put it, "government red tape" has interfered with patients' right to save their lives.[35] Yet critics predict that right-to-try laws will have little impact on access.

In the Abigail Burroughs and other high-profile cases it was drug companies, not FDA officials, who blocked patients' access to experimental drugs.[36] Because right-to-try laws don't require drug companies to comply with patients' compassionate-use requests, the laws do nothing to help with the real access problem. Indeed, removing the FDA from the process could actually make things worse. Officials at the FDA often help patients and physicians negotiate with drug companies about compassionate use.[37] Without FDA involvement, fewer companies might be willing to supply patients with experimental drugs.

Right-to-try critics also point out that many patients have received experimental drugs through the FDA system.[38] When companies say no to patient requests, FDA access regulations are not the reason. Because the companies' overriding goal is to gain FDA approval of their drugs, they want to devote their limited resources to conducting the research that will make approval possible. Producing drugs for patients outside trials can be costly to companies.[39] Even though the FDA permits them to recover their costs, companies may be unable to manage the logistics involved in operating a large compassionate-use program.

Opponents say right-to-try laws will not change this situation. They also warn that the FDA could challenge unauthorized drug distribution as a violation of federal law.[40] Companies distributing drugs without FDA permission could damage their efforts to win FDA approval of those drugs too. It isn't surprising that drug company lobbyists have "serious concerns with any approach to make investigational medicines available that seeks to bypass the oversight of the Food and Drug Administration and clinical trial process."[41] Drug companies would be acting against their self-interest if they provided drugs outside the FDA's compassionate-use program.

A further problem is that right-to-try laws fail to address existing inequities in compassionate access to experimental drugs. Under right-to-try laws, access would continue to be available only to patients whose doctors are energetic and savvy enough to convince companies to provide the drugs. And right-to-try laws, like FDA regulations, allow companies to charge patients for drugs. This means that only patients who can afford the charges would gain access. As the mother of a patient seeking access complained, right-to-try laws "ignore the elephant in the room, which is cost."[42]

HOW ACCESS AFFECTS PATIENTS

Right-to-try advocates say that liberal access is the best approach for patients. They tell stories of patients helped by experimental drugs as well as stories of patients who suffered and died without them. Advocates work with patients and their families to publicize these compelling accounts.

But access advocates leave out other kinds of patient stories. They leave out stories of patients who tried experimental measures but paid a price for doing so. Rather than giving patients longer or more comfortable lives, those measures hastened death and increased suffering. Right-to-try advocates also leave out stories showing that wide patient access can make it harder to complete the studies needed to determine whether experimental approaches are truly beneficial. These stories show that liberal access is not always the pro-patient position it purports to be.

Stories in the Access Debate

Patients' stories are a staple of right-to-try campaigns. Most famous is the story of Abigail Burroughs—a college student whose head-and-neck cancer failed to respond to standard therapies. Burroughs wanted to try two experimental drugs that were being studied at the time. But patients with the type of cancer she had weren't eligible for the studies, and the drug companies refused to grant her compassionate-use request. Burroughs died when she was just twenty-one years old. One of the drugs she wanted to try was later approved to treat head-and-neck cancer. Her father, founder of the Abigail Alliance, is convinced that she would have survived if she had been able to obtain the drug.[43]

Right-to-try advocates have further distressing stories to tell. The Goldwater Institute's right-to-try proposal begins with the story of Kianna Karnes, a nurse and mother of four who died of kidney cancer the very day that the

FDA and two drug companies agreed to cooperate with her compassionate-use request. The proposal concludes with the plea of another terminally ill patient who claimed she was denied an experimental drug because the manufacturer was afraid of "a government hassle."[44]

Stories have played a central role in legislative hearings on right-to-try laws. The lead sponsor of Missouri's bill was Jim Neely, a physician-legislator whose stepdaughter had been diagnosed with advanced colon cancer. His stepdaughter wasn't eligible for any clinical trials, but she still wanted to try experimental drugs. Neely and two other men with children in similar situations told their stories at a legislative hearing on the bill, which was unanimously approved in 2014.[45] (The right-to-try law didn't help Neely's stepdaughter obtain the drugs she sought, however, and she died the following year.[46])

Another patient's story helped persuade Colorado's legislature to pass a right-to-try law. One of the law's most vocal supporters was the wife of Nick Auden, a patient who died of melanoma after failing to convince two drug companies to provide him with promising experimental drugs. Although the companies said their decisions were based on safety concerns and an inadequate drug supply, Auden's wife blamed the FDA for the refusal.[47]

As one journalist put it, the "frustration of tragedy" drives right-to-try supporters. Some are people "motivated to honor ones they have lost to illness"; others are "racing to save sick family who are still living."[48] They are people who have seen one side of the compassionate-use situation, and this experience shapes their access position.

But right-to-try advocates aren't the only ones with tragic stories to tell. Law professor Michael Malinowski tells a tragic story about his father, who had terminal cancer and "aggressively sought and received ... experimental treatments—from drugs to a series of surgeries." The drugs, however, "worsened his health immediately; the side effects were horrific."[49] For the remaining months of his life, Malinowski's father was on high doses of morphine for pain. He lost more than a hundred pounds before he died.

Malinowski believes his father was "in a state of denial" about his impending death, a denial that no doctor was willing to confront. Doctors were eager to provide his father with experimental measures, but none brought up the palliative-care options that could have increased his comfort and extended his life. In Malinowski's father's case, experimental interventions led to a painful and distressing death rather than a longer and better life.[50]

Former cancer patient Musa Mayer tells another instructive story about the downsides of access. During the 1990s, Mayer worked to help two women with advanced breast cancer gain access to an experimental treatment that combined high-dose chemotherapy with bone marrow transplantation. The treatment was supported by phase 2 trial evidence but had not been evaluated in phase 3 trials. The chemotherapy drugs used in the treatment had been approved, so the FDA's compassionate-use rules did not apply in this case.[51] But many insurers were unwilling to cover the experimental treatment. In this campaign, insurance companies were the target of compassionate-use claims.

Despite a lack of solid evidence on safety and effectiveness, many women wanted to try the combination of high-dose chemotherapy and bone marrow transplantation. They wanted to "go out fighting" and show their families they had done everything to survive.[52] But the women Mayer helped did not have good outcomes. One had a fatal hemorrhage soon after her bone marrow transplant, and treatment side effects led to the other woman's death. After that, Mayer wrote, "I finally understood what later seemed obvious—that there were other voices we had not been listening for being drowned out by the clamor for access, the voices of those who had died from the treatment itself."[53]

Mayer realized that the compassionate-access campaign was neglecting other voices too. There were the "voices of those women who suffered from temporary or permanent disabilities as a result of their transplants." There were the voices of women whose cancer progressed despite the treatment. And there were the voices of women "whose future treatments for advanced disease had been compromised by the massive doses of chemotherapy they had already endured." Many of these women kept quiet about their situations, because they did not want "to demoralize the others, or second guess their own choices."[54]

Women who wanted the unproven breast cancer treatment were often able to obtain it without enrolling in research. As a result, it took many years to conduct randomized clinical trials evaluating its risks and benefits. Women who wanted to try the treatment were unwilling to take the chance of being assigned to standard treatment, which had low success rates. But when the research was finally completed, the findings showed that the experimental treatment was no better than the standard treatment.

Mayer sees history repeating itself in recent compassionate-use campaigns. "With legal liability off the table, FDA out of the picture, and the efficacy bar lowered as far as it will go," she asks, "how long would it take to reach the first disaster relating to drug toxicity? How many savings accounts would be emptied in the vain pursuit of hope?"[55]

Physician Darshak Sanghavi is worried about compassionate use too. To explain his concerns, he tells the stories of two patients. One was Sarah Broom, a thirty-five-year-old mother of three with advanced lung cancer. She lived in New Zealand but was an Oxford University graduate with influential friends around the world. Through her connections, she was able to locate and participate in a drug study. She did well for two years; then her tumors began growing again. Her last hope was to try a different experimental drug, but the drug company turned down her request for compassionate use. Broom and her doctor refused to give up, however, and company officials eventually agreed to give her the drug. She lived another year before finally succumbing to cancer.[56]

Experimental drugs gave Sarah Broom a few valuable years with her family—years in which she felt well and could enjoy her remaining life. But for the second patient whose story Sanghavi tells—his own father—access to an experimental measure was disastrous. In Sanghavi's father's case, an insurance company agreed to cover the costs of an expensive, FDA-approved drug that had not been fully evaluated in patients with his illness, a fatal condition called idiopathic pulmonary fibrosis. The only evidence came from a small preliminary study in which nine patients with the condition had shown substantial improvement after receiving the drug.[57]

Sadly, those early study results were misleading. Injections of the drug did not help Sanghavi's father. Instead, they "caused raging fevers that left him confined to bed in terrible pain." A few years later, results from a larger and more rigorous study showed that the drug was both ineffective and risky for patients with idiopathic pulmonary fibrosis, triggering lung infections in the patients who took it.[58] Sanghavi believes "[i]t would have been better if my father never took it. And because we had found a backdoor way of getting it—he never joined any study—no drug company or regulator learned anything constructive from his death."[59]

Taken altogether, the stories above reveal the different sides of so-called compassionate use. No single story can present a full picture of patients' interests in the access debate. Access gives some patients the relief they are seeking, but leaves others with shorter lives and more suffering. As these stories show, patients' freedom to try experimental measures is at best a mixed blessing.

Empirical Data on Patients' Experiences

Patients' stories are graphic and powerful, conveying the real urgency, joy, and misery surrounding the quest to obtain experimental drugs. Empirical studies are another source of information relevant to compassionate-use policy. Researchers have explored patients' experiences with and beliefs about experimental drugs through interviews, surveys, and other methods. Not enough of these studies have been done, but those that exist offer insights that belong in the right-to-try debate.

A study published in 2007 is one example. Acting on their belief that "patients' views and experiences should inform the debate about the appropriate way to provide access to investigational agents,"[60] a research team asked one hundred terminally ill patients for their views on such access. The patients surveyed were hoping to participate in an early human study of a widely publicized cancer drug that was in short supply.[61]

In their survey responses, patients most often endorsed two criteria for deciding who should have access to experimental drugs when supplies are limited. The patients preferred these drugs to be made available to (1) patients with the greatest need or most chance of benefit and (2) patients in studies, because research would produce the best information about drug safety and effectiveness. Few of the surveyed patients thought that experimental drugs should go to any patient who wanted them. At the same time, a majority thought it was too hard for patients to get access to the drugs. They also thought that "knowing the right people" and "being persistent" would increase a patient's access chances.

Patients responding to this survey sympathized with terminally ill individuals seeking access, but they also recognized the public's interest in preserving a research system that can detect which new agents are truly safe and effective. As the study authors observed, the patients' responses "reflect the core ethical tension between maximizing scientific advancement and making investigational agents available to ailing individuals."[62] Most patients believed in a right to access, but they also supported rules that prioritize certain patients over others and take into account the public's interest in a rigorous drug evaluation system.

Other studies have considered the quality of terminally ill patients' decisions to participate in drug trials. Most of these patients have the same mindset as patients seeking experimental drugs outside trials—they are hoping that a novel drug will be more effective than existing treatments. Despite strict requirements for information disclosure and informed consent in research, study after study shows that many subjects overestimate the chance that experimental drugs will help them and underestimate the drugs' potential to cause harm. Some subjects don't understand that the trials' primary purpose is to produce knowledge, not to provide the best treatment to individual trial subjects.[63] Others realize that drug trials often fail to benefit subjects, yet remain unrealistically optimistic about their own chances. Contrary to the objective evidence, they believe they have a "greater likelihood of experiencing positive outcomes or avoiding negative outcomes compared with others in the same or similar situation."[64]

Researchers have also found that social expectations lead some patients to try experimental drugs. In one interview study, a majority of subjects enrolled in cancer trials said they expected a therapeutic benefit from their participation, and more than a third of the subjects said their optimism was related to the expectations of others.[65] Some linked optimism to their duty to "reassure or help loved ones in dealing with the patient's own struggle with cancer."[66] The problem is that patients' loved ones may have the same unrealistic hopes that patients have. Studies have shown that even doctors and researchers may overestimate the chance that experimental drugs will benefit patients.[67]

Studies about patients' experiences while they are taking experimental drugs are relevant to access policy too. One such study involved in-depth interviews with advanced-cancer patients who had participated in early-phase drug trials. As the trials progressed, the patients reported feeling more and more burdened by the experience. Some of the burdens were related to the trials, such as the extra hospital visits and tests required to gather study data. But patients were also burdened by the side effects of the drugs—side effects that they had not anticipated. Over time these patients developed "a feeling that the harm was too great, and a sense of disillusionment with what was on offer took over."[68] The majority of these patients had to leave the trial because they had severe side effects or cancer progression. Most said they did not regret their earlier choice to participate, however, for it had given them a chance to help themselves and others.

Studies like these shed light on terminally ill patients' experiences with experimental drugs, but there are not enough such studies. Many terminally ill subjects in drug trials have disappointing results, but researchers have rarely looked into their experiences. Indeed, one team that wanted to interview cancer trial participants with poor outcomes was blocked by a research ethics committee worried about the burdens that interviews would impose on those participants.[69]

Without data from patients who have had poor outcomes in experimental trials, we will have an incomplete picture of how access affects patients. In the case described above, the ethics committee's desire to protect trial participants with poor outcomes was understandable, but it might have been misguided. One review found that a majority of terminally ill patients had positive attitudes about participating in research on end-of-life care.[70] It is likely that some trial participants with poor outcomes would be willing and able to discuss their experiences with researchers.

Also missing from the access picture is information about patients receiving experimental drugs outside trials. Since the 1980s, thousands of terminally ill patients have tried drugs through the FDA's compassionate-use program. To my knowledge, no one has taken an in-depth look at what happened to them. How many patients had their lives lengthened or improved? How many experienced toxic side effects that made them feel worse? How many died as a result of those side effects? How many regretted their choice to try the drugs? We ought to know much more about how patients as well as their families evaluate compassionate access.[71]

TOWARD A MORE REPRESENTATIVE PICTURE OF PATIENT EXPERIENCES

Right-to-try advocates claim they are on a mission of mercy, seeking to give more terminally ill patients a last opportunity to postpone mortality. Time will tell whether right-to-try laws have any real impact on access to experimental drugs. At this point, it's far from certain that patients in right-to-try states will succeed in obtaining drugs without FDA permission.[72] And if the laws do enable more patients to try the drugs, it is unlikely that many will benefit.

Going forward, the right-to-try debate should be more informed than it has been. People ought to receive a realistic description of what happens to patients who succeed in gaining access to experimental drugs. They should hear stories about the many patients whose conditions don't respond to experimental drugs as well as stories about the patients who suffer and die sooner because they tried the drugs. The selective storytelling that has dominated campaigns in support of the right to try presents a distorted picture, contributing to policies that could actually disserve patients.

A more accurate picture of patients' experiences could produce better decisions about right-to-try laws. It could also help patients and families see the limits and drawbacks of trying drugs whose effects are largely unknown. A more accurate picture of patients' experiences could influence access advocacy too. It could encourage advocates to address the broad interests of terminally ill patients and their families through programs that focus less on improbable treatment outcomes and more on patients' common medical and social needs.

The right-to-try campaign may be a small policy development, but it raises fundamental questions about our nation's attitudes toward death and dying. Right-to-try laws portray experimental treatments as desirable, even optimal, responses to life-threatening illness. A wider look at patients' experiences could reveal the human costs of this approach, drawing attention to policies and programs that could offer help that is more meaningful to people near the end of their lives.

NOTES

1. See Darcy Olsen, "Dying Patients Should Have 'Right to Try' New Treatments," *Time*, November 10, 2015. Retrieved December 30, 2015, from http://time.com/4091290/right-to-try.
2. Musa Mayer, "When Clinical Trials Are Compromised: A Perspective from a Patient Advocate," *PLoS Medicine* 2 (2005): 1060–62, 1062. Physician Louise Aronson believes that medical and research professionals should make more use of stories when they discuss science and medicine with the public. She writes that "a single well-told story of human suffering trumps the most eloquent explanation of a large-scale trial." Louise Aronson, "Story as Evidence, Evidence as Story," *Journal of the American Medical Association* 314 (2015): 125–26.
3. See Abigail Alliance for Better Access to Developmental Drugs v. von Eschenbach, 445 F.3d 470, 482 (D.C. Cir. 2006).
4. For a general review of the process, see US Food and Drug Administration, "The FDA's Drug Review Process: Ensuring

Drugs Are Safe and Effective." Retrieved May 6, 2015, from http://www.fda.gov/drugs/resourcesforyou/consumers/ucm143534.htm.

5. "Overview of Clinical Trials," CenterWatch. Retrieved May 6, 2015, from http://www.centerwatch.com/clinical-trials/overview.aspx.

6. Gregory Petsko, "When Failure Should Be the Option," *BMC Biology* 8 (2010): 1–3, 2.

7. J. DiMasi et al., "Trends in Risks Associated with New Drug Development: Success Rates for Investigational Drugs," *Clinical Pharmacology & Therapeutics* 87 (2010): 272–77.

8. Michael Hay et al., "Clinical Development Success Rates for Investigational Drugs," *Nature Biotechnology* 32 (2014): 40–51.

9. See Manish Agrawal and Ezekiel J. Emanuel, "Ethics of Phase 1 Oncology Studies," *Journal of the American Medical Association* 290 (2003): 1075–82, which describes approved cancer drugs that have low success rates in patients. See also Benjamin P. Falit and Cary P. Gross, "Access to Experimental Drugs for Terminally Ill Patients," *Journal of the American Medical Association* 300 (2008): 2793–95, 2793, which observes that "only a fraction" of patients receiving approved cancer drugs experience a health benefit.

10. See Julie Brintnall-Karabelas et al., "Improving Recruitment in Clinical Trials: Why Eligible Participants Decline," *Journal of Empirical Research on Human Research Ethics* 6, no. 1 (2011): 69–74; Manik Chahal, "Off-Trial Access to Experimental Cancer Agents for the Terminally Ill: Balancing the Needs of Individuals and Society," *Journal of Medical Ethics* 36 (2010): 367–70.

11. "Investigational New Drug, Antibiotic, and Biological Drug Product Regulations; Treatment Use and Sale," 52 *Fed. Reg.* 19,476–77 (May 22, 1987).

12. "Our Story," Abigail Alliance for Better Access to Developmental Drugs. Retrieved May 15, 2015, from http://www.abigail-alliance.org/story.php.

13. Judy Foreman, "Dying Patient's Fight to Access Trial Drugs Met with Resistance," *Baltimore Sun*, September 29, 2003. Retrieved May 15, 2015, from http://

articles.baltimoresun.com/2003-09-29/news/0309290141_1_experimental-drugs-abigail-burroughs-new-drugs.

14. For details on the court cases, see Rebecca Dresser, "The 'Right to Try' Investigational Drugs: Science and Stories in the Access Debate," *Texas Law Review* 93 (2015): 1631–57.

15. "Expanded Access to Investigational Drugs for Treatment Use," 74 *Fed. Reg.* 40, 900 (Aug. 13, 2009). The regulations still do not allow companies to profit from providing investigational drugs. Code of Federal Regulations 21 (2014): § 312.8(c).

16. See "Expanded Access," 40,912–13, which argues for "flexibility in the evidentiary standards" applied to individual patient requests and notes that treatment use of unapproved drugs "may be sought quite early in a drug's development, and at any point during the development."

17. Christina Corieri, "Everyone Deserves the Right to Try: Empowering the Terminally Ill to Take Control of Their Treatment," February 11, 2014. Retrieved May 12, 2015, from http://goldwaterinstitute.org/en/work/topics/health-care/right-to-try/everyone-deserves-right-try-empowering-terminally-/.

18. For texts of specific state laws and bills, see Alexander Gaffnet, " 'Right to Try' Legislative Tracker," June 24, 2015. Retrieved December 30, 2015, from http://www.raps.org/Regulatory-Focus/News/Databases/2015/06/24/21133/Right-to-Try-Legislation-Tracker/.

19. Ibid.

20. David Gorski, " 'Right to Try' Laws and *Dallas Buyers' Club*: Great Movie, Terrible for Patients and Terrible Policy," March 8, 2014. Retrieved May 12, 2015, from http://www.sciencebasedmedicine.org/right-to-try-laws-and-dallas-buyers-club-great-movie-terrible-public-policy/.

21. It's hard to see how practicing physicians could make good decisions about early-phase drugs when so little is known about their safety and effectiveness. See David W. Borhani and J. Adam Butts, "Rethinking Clinical Trials: Biology's Mysteries," *Science* 334 (2011): 1346–47, which questions whether doctors should prescribe "unproven drugs . . . when faced with volumes of uncertain data."

22. Corieri, "Everyone Deserves." For examples of these arguments, see Les Halpin et al., "Improving Access to Medicines: Empowering Patients in the Quest to Improve Treatment for Rare Lethal Diseases," *Journal of Medical Ethics* 41 (2015): 987-89; Eugene Volokh, "Medical Self-Defense, Prohibited Experimental Therapies, and Payment for Organs," *Harvard Law Review* 120 (2007): 1813–46; John A. Robertson, "Controversial Medical Treatment and the Right to Health Care," *Hastings Center Report* 36, no. 6 (2006): 15–20; Vicki Brower, "Food and Drug Administration Responds to Pressure for Expanded Drug Access," *Journal of the National Cancer Institute* 106 (June 11, 2014): 1–9; Simon Woods and Pauline McCormack, "Disputing the Ethics of Research: The Challenge from Bioethics and Patient Activism to the Interpretation of the Declaration of Helsinki in Clinical Trials," *Bioethics* 27 (2013): 243–50; Chahal, "Off-Trial Access."

23. See Elizabeth Richardson, "Right-to-Try Laws (Updated)," *Health Policy Briefs*, April 9, 2015. Retrieved May 20, 2015, from http://www.healthaffairs.org/healthpolicybriefs/brief.php?brief_id=136. Richardson reports that in the four years preceding her report, the FDA received almost six thousand applications and granted all but thirty-three of them. See also Kelly Servick, "'Right to Try' Laws Bypass FDA for Last-Ditch Treatments," *Science* 344 (2014): 1329, which reports that the FDA received almost one thousand access requests in 2013 and denied only three. In an interview, one FDA official said he could remember just one access denial, a case in which parents had refused standard cancer treatment for their child. See Jerome Groopman, "The Right to a Trial," *New Yorker* (December 18, 2006). Retrieved May 12, 2015, from http://www.newyorker.com/magazine/2006/12/18/the-right-to-a-trial.

24. Corieri, "Everyone Deserves." Until recently, the FDA used a submission form that demanded extensive information from physicians and sponsors requesting access. But in February 2015, in "an effort to streamline the submission process for individual patient expanded access," the agency proposed a much simplified form that officials estimated would take

about forty-five minutes to complete. See *Draft Guidance, Individual Patient Expanded Access Applications: Form FDA 3926*, February 10, 2015. Retrieved May 21, 2015, from www. fda.gov/downloads/drugs/guidancecomplianceregulatoryin-formation/guidances/ucm432717.pdf.

25. See Gorski, "'Right to Try' Laws."

26. Ibid.

27. Michael J. Malinowski, "Throwing Dirt on Doctor Franken-stein's Grave: Access to Experimental Treatments at the End of Life," *Hastings Law Journal* 65 (2014): 615–51, 657. See also George J. Annas, "The Changing Landscape of Human Experimentation: Nuremberg, Helsinki, and Beyond," *Health Matrix* 2 (1992): 119–40, which argues for strict limits on re-search participation for terminally ill patients.

28. Chahal, "Off-Trial Access," 368. See also Victoria Weisfeld et al., *Public Engagement and Clinical Trials: New Models and Disruptive Technologies* (Washington, DC: National Academies Press, 2012), 2, which identifies "the increasing difficulty of recruiting and retaining an appropriate human subject population for specific clinical trials" as a "significant problem."

29. Code of Federal Regulations 21 (2014): § 312.305(a)(3). The FDA treatment access regulations require doctors to report information about adverse events to drug companies and the FDA. The reporting requirements promote public health by strengthening the evidentiary basis for approval decisions. Right-to-try laws fail to include such reporting requirements.

30. Volokh, "Medical Self-Defense," note 81. Some access sup-porters think the public health threat has been exagger-ated. See Robertson, "Controversial Medical Treatment," 17. Other access supporters argue that regulators should speed up the drug approval process by adopting alternative meth-ods of collecting evidence about new drugs. See Michael Keane, "It's Time for Change," *Journal of Medical Ethics* 41 (2014): 954–55.

31. See Seema Shah and Patricia Zettler, "From a Constitutional Right to a Policy of Exceptions: Abigail Alliance and the Future of Access to Experimental Therapy," *Yale Journal of*

Health Policy, Law, and Ethics 10 (2010): 135–96; Elizabeth Weeks Leonard, "The Public's Right to Health: When Patient Rights Threaten the Commons," *Washington University Law Review* 86 (2009): 1335–96. Colorado's right-to-try law limits investigational-drug access to patients who have "been unable to participate in a clinical trial for the terminal illness within one hundred miles of the patient's home address . . . or not been accepted to the clinical trial within one week of completion of the clinical trial application process." Colorado Revised Statutes Annotated § 25-45-103(1)(a)(III) (West Supp. 2014). Other right-to-try laws don't include these restrictions.

32. Leonard, "Public's Right to Health," 1384.
33. Brower, "Food and Drug Administration," 2.
34. See Leonard, "Public's Right to Health," 1386–87; Shah and Zettler, "From a Constitutional Right," 194–95. See also Carter Snead, "Unenumerated Rights and the Limits of Analogy: A Critique of the Right to Medical Self-Defense," *Harvard Law Review Forum* 121 (2007): 1–11, 11, which notes that there is "no history or tradition of courts privileging the preferences of patients (including those suffering from terminal illnesses) for a particular prohibited medical intervention over governmental concerns about public health."
35. Eleanor Clift, "The '*Dallas Buyers Club*' Bill," *Daily Beast*, March 4, 2014. Retrieved May 17, 2015, from http://www.the-dailybeast.com/articles/2014/03/04/the-dallas-buyers-club-bill.html.
36. See Jerry Menikoff, "Beyond *Abigail Alliance*: The Reality Behind the Right to Get Investigational Drugs," *University of Kansas Law Review* 56 (2008): 1045–74, 1059–60, which notes that none of the four plaintiffs in the Abigail Alliance case showed that the FDA interfered with their access efforts. See also Brady Dennis and Ariana Eunjung Cha, "'Right to Try' Laws Spur Debate over Dying Patients' Access to Experimental Drugs," *Washington Post*, May 16, 2014. Retrieved May 17, 2015, from http://www.washingtonpost.com/national/health-science/right-to-try-laws-spur-debate-over-dying-patients-access-to-experimental-drugs/2014/05/16/820e08c8-dcfa-11e3-b745-87d39690c5c0_story.html;

David Kroll, "The False Hope of Colorado's 'Right to Try' Investigational Drug Law," *Forbes*, May 19, 2014. Retrieved May 17, 2015, from http://www.forbes.com/sites/davidkroll/2014/05/19/the-false-hope-of-colorados-right-to-try-act/.

37. *The Diane Rehm Show*, "Debate over 'Right-to-Try' Laws," May 27, 2014. Retrieved May 17, 2015, from http://thedianerehm-show.org/shows/2014-05-27/debate-over-right-try-laws/transcript. See also Ariana Eunjung Cha, "Crowdsourcing Medical Decisions: Ethicists Worry Josh Hardy Case May Set Bad Precedent," *Washington Post*, March 23, 2014. Retrieved May 17, 2015, from http://www.washingtonpost.com/national/health-science/crowdsourcing-medical-decisions-ethicists-worry-josh-hardy-case-may-set-bad-precedent/2014/03/23/f8591446-ab81-11e3-adbc-888c8010c799_story.html.

38. For discussion of the potential business and public relations advantages for companies providing access, see Brower, "Food and Drug Administration"; Cha, "Crowdsourcing Medical Decisions."

39. See Brower, "Food and Drug Administration"; Arthur L. Caplan, "Why 'Right to Try' Laws Won't Help Desperately Ill Patients," *Medscape*, June 19, 2014. Retrieved May 17, 2015, from http://www.medscape.com/viewarticle/826708. Companies also worry that negative effects detected in patients could make the FDA more cautious about approving an investigational drug, although agency officials say this fear is unfounded. Servick, "'Right to Try' Laws"; *The Diane Rehm Show*, "Debate over 'Right to Try' Laws."

40. See Patricia J. Zettler and Henry T. Greely, "The Strange Allure of State 'Right-to-Try' Laws," *JAMA Internal Medicine* 174 (2014): 1885–86, which notes that federal law trumps state law.

41. John Tozzi, "Do Dying Patients Have a Right to Try Experimental Drugs? Libertarians Say Yes," *Businessweek*, August 21, 2014. Retrieved May 17, 2015, from http://www.bloomberg.com/bw/articles/2014-08-21/do-dying-patients-have-a-right-to-try-experimental-drugs-libertarians-say-yes.

42. Mary Lou Byrd, "Third State Passes 'Right to Try' Legislation," *Washington Free Beacon*, July 17, 2014. Retrieved May 17,

2015, from http://freebeacon.com/issues/third-state-passes-right-to-try-legislation/.
43. Byrd, "Third State."
44. Corieri, "Everyone Deserves." The first federal bill promoting liberal access was nicknamed "Kianna's Law." See Groopman, "Right to a Trial."
45. *PBS NewsHour,* " 'Right to Try' Law Gives Terminal Patients Access to Drugs Not Approved by FDA," June 21, 2014. Retrieved May 18, 2015, from http://www.pbs.org/newshour/bb/right-try-law-gives-terminal-patients-access-non-fda-approved-drugs/; Mike Sherry, "Missouri Becomes Third State to Enact 'Right to Try' Drug Law," October 8, 2014. Retrieved May 18, 2015, from http://kbia.org/post/missouri-becomes-third-state-enact-right-try-drug-law; Virginia Young, "Missouri Could Join Push for Experimental Drugs for Terminally Ill," *St. Louis Post-Dispatch,* June 3, 2014. Retrieved May 18, 2015, from http://www.stltoday.com/news/local/govt-and-politics/missouri-could-join-push-for-experimental-drugs-for-terminally-ill/article_c213ab2a-9612-5661-8d75-951c84c271eb.html.
46. Michele Munz, "Missouri's 'Right to Try' Law No Guarantee Patient Will Get Experimental Drugs," *St. Louis Post-Dispatch,* May 20, 2015. Retrieved May 21, 2015, from http://www.stltoday.com/news/local/metro/missouri-s-right-to-try-law-no-guarantee-patient-will/article_05c07958-5217-5c3f-9f15-1a43c8a3e740.html.
47. Kurtis Lee, " 'Right to Try' Aims to Limit Bureaucracy for Colorado's Terminally Ill," *Denver Post,* April 1, 2014. Retrieved May 18, 2015, from http://www.denverpost.com/politics/ci_25463368/right-try-aims-limit-bureaucracy-colorados-terminally-ill.
48. Amity Shlaes, "The Right to Try," *National Review,* May 14, 2014. Retrieved May 18, 2015, from http://www.nationalreview.com/article/377907/right-try-amity-shlaes.
49. Malinowski, "Throwing Dirt," 618.
50. Ibid., 616–19. See also Jennifer S. Temel et al., "Early Palliative Care for Patients with Metastatic Non-small-cell Lung Cancer," *New England Journal of Medicine* 363 (2010): 733–42, which found that early use of palliative care extended patients' survival by approximately two months and resulted

in "clinically meaningful improvements in quality of life and mood" compared with standard care.

51. Once a drug is approved for one medical use, doctors may prescribe it for other, "off-label" uses. Doctors sometimes prescribe cancer drugs off label without good evidence that the drugs are safe and effective for the off-label application. Erika P. Hamilton et al., "Availability of Experimental Therapy outside Oncology Randomized Clinical Trials in the United States," *Journal of Clinical Oncology* 28 (2010): 5067–73.

52. Mayer, "When Clinical Trials," 1060–61.

53. Musa Mayer, "Listen to All the Voices: An Advocate's Perspective on Early Access to Investigational Therapies," *Clinical Trials* 3 (2006): 149–53, 150.

54. Ibid.

55. Ibid., 151.

56. Darshak M. Sanghavi, "The Pills of Last Resort: How Dying Patients Get Access to Experimental Drugs," *New York Times Magazine*, October 31, 2013. Retrieved May 18, 2015, from http://www.nytimes.com/2013/11/03/magazine/how-dying-patients-get-access-to-experimental-drugs.html.

57. Rolf Ziesche et al., "A Preliminary Study of Long-Term Treatment with Interferon Gamma-1b and Low-Dose Prednisolone in Patients with Idiopathic Pulmonary Fibrosis," *New England Journal of Medicine* 341 (1999): 1264–69.

58. Ganesh Raghu et al., "A Placebo-Controlled Trial of Interferon Gamma-1b in Patients with Idiopathic Pulmonary Fibrosis," *New England Journal of Medicine* 350 (2004): 125–33.

59. Sanghavi, "Pills of Last Resort." A news story reported that a high-ranking FDA official's wife "suffered terribly" when she obtained access to an unapproved drug through enrollment in a clinical trial. She experienced several toxic reactions to the drug, including swelling of the heart, soaring blood pressure, and severe fatigue. Gardiner Harris, "F.D.A. Regulator, Widowed by Cancer, Helps Speed Drug Approval," *New York Times*, January 2, 2016. Retrieved January 5, 2016, from http://nyti.ms/1OOY5BD. For more stories of patients who fared well and badly after obtaining access to investigational drugs, see Groopman, "Right to a Trial."

60. Rebecca D. Pentz et al., "Who Should Go First in Trials with Scarce Agents?," *IRB: Ethics & Human Research* 29, no. 4 (2007): 1–6.

61. Later phase 2 trials found that the drug, called endostatin, had very little effect on patients' tumors. See Ariel Whitworth, "Endostatin: Are We Waiting for Godot?," *Journal of the National Cancer Institute* 98 (2006): 731–35.

62. Pentz et al., "Who Should Go First," 4.

63. This misunderstanding, known as the "therapeutic misconception," has been widely observed. For example, one study team conducting surveys and interviews found that nearly 70 percent of participants in phase 1 cancer trials could not correctly answer questions about the purpose of trials and how treatment is chosen in trials. Rebecca D. Pentz et al., "Therapeutic Misconception, Misestimation, and Optimism in Participants Enrolled in Phase 1 Trials," *Cancer* 118 (2012): 4571–78.

64. Joshua Crites and Eric Kodish, "Unrealistic Optimism and the Ethics of Phase I Cancer Research," *Journal of Medical Ethics* 39 (2013): 403–6, 404. See also Don Swekoski and Deborah Barnbaum, "The Gambler's Fallacy, the Therapeutic Misconception, and Unrealistic Optimism," *IRB: Ethics & Human Research* 35, no. 2 (2013): 1–6, which describes how patients' lack of understanding or acceptance of low chance of benefit interferes with informed consent.

65. Daniel P. Sulmasy et al., "The Culture of Faith and Hope: Patients' Justifications for Their High Estimations of Expected Therapeutic Benefit When Enrolling in Early Phase Oncology Trials," *Cancer* 116 (2010): 3702–11, 3707.

66. Ibid., 3705.

67. See, for example, Victoria Miller et al., "Hope and Persuasion by Physicians during Informed Consent," *Journal of Clinical Oncology* 32 (2014): 3229–35; Christopher Daugherty et al., "Perceptions of Cancer Patients and Their Physicians Involved in Phase I Trials," *Journal of Clinical Oncology* 13 (1995): 1062–72.

68. Karen Cox, "Enhancing Cancer Clinical Trial Management: Recommendations from a Qualitative Study of Trial Participants' Experiences," *Psycho-Oncology* 9 (2000): 314–22, 317.

69. S. M. Madsen et al., "Participating in a Cancer Clinical Trial? The Balancing of Options in the Loneliness of Autonomy: A Grounded Theory Interview Study," *Acta Oncologica* 46 (2007): 49–59.

70. Marjolein H. Gysels et al., "Patient, Caregiver, Health Professional and Researcher Views and Experiences of Participating in Research at the End of Life: A Critical Interpretive Synthesis of the Literature," *BMC Medical Research Methodology* 12 (2012): 1–17.

71. In 2014, a group that included drug company leaders, FDA officials, bioethicists, and a patient advocate urged companies to create registries tracking outcomes in patients receiving treatment access to investigational drugs. Darshak Sanghavi, Meaghan George, and Sara Bencic, "Individual Patient Expanded Access: Developing Principles for a Structural and Regulatory Framework," *Health Affairs Blog*, July 31, 2014. Retrieved May 24, 2015, from http://healthaffairs.org/blog/2014/07/31/individual-patient-expanded-access-developing-principles-for-a-structural-and-regulatory-framework/.

72. An October 2015 survey identified no cases in which state right-to-try laws helped patients to obtain investigational drugs without FDA authorization. Steven Ross Johnson, "Despite Political Support, State Right-to-Try Laws Show No Takeup," *Modern Healthcare*, October 17, 2015. Retrieved December 30, 2015, from http://www.modernhealthcare.com/article/20151017/MAGAZINE/310179969.

7

Embedded Ethics
in Developing-Country
Research

■□■

IN 2015, government agencies and other organizations were gearing up for clinical trials to test potential vaccines for the Ebola virus. To plan the trials, researchers and health officials from the United States and other wealthy nations joined with their counterparts in the African countries hit hardest by the disease. But trial planners faced many challenges, including public mistrust.

Two *New York Times* journalists reported that mistrust was threatening subject recruitment in Liberia, the site of one proposed trial. The journalists quoted a Liberian man who believed the Ebola virus was created by people in the United States. The man said, "So why didn't they do this trial in America, but they decide to come to Liberia?" On Liberian radio, a reporter asked whether signing a trial consent form would be equivalent to signing a "death warrant." A local news story declared, "Liberians are not animals."[1]

Besides recruitment problems, planners faced doubts about their ability to protect trial volunteers who developed fevers or other vaccine side effects. In Guinea, another trial location, critics said that some treatment centers weren't equipped to deliver high-quality care to volunteers. Monitoring volunteers for side effects would also be difficult, for people in villages moved around and couldn't always be easily located.[2] Settling on a proper payment for volunteers was a struggle too. As the *Times* journalists reported, some US researchers questioned the lead Liberian researcher's proposal to pay volunteers the equivalent of $30 for each trial visit, a sum much higher than many local residents could earn in a day.

Recognizing that "social mobilization" would be essential to the success of the trials, planners worked with communities to respond to these problems.[3] They developed consent forms and recruitment materials that took local circumstances into account. They asked communities to choose a local resident to be in charge of reporting side effects that trial subjects experienced between scheduled study visits. They gave the designated reporters cell phones to allow quick access to study teams. After the Liberian researcher defended his payment proposal as reasonable compensation for volunteers' travel costs and lost wages, other planners agreed to it.[4]

The issues faced by the planners of the Ebola vaccine trials are not unusual in global health research. Much of this research is financially supported and initiated by people from wealthy countries but carried out in developing countries, where local residents serve as research subjects. In this context, factors like mistrust, poverty, and low literacy can have major impacts on the conduct of health research.

SUBJECT PERSPECTIVES IN DEVELOPING-COUNTRY RESEARCH

The settings of developing-country research are quite diverse. Subjects' experiences, as well as the relevant research ethics issues, vary a great deal. If the material I describe in this chapter shows anything, it shows that the specific context of research strongly influences the ethics of that research. "Attending to particularity" is required in evaluations of research ethics wherever they occur.[5]

While subjects in developing-country research do report many experiences that resemble those of study subjects in wealthy nations, social conditions also can have a big impact on their experiences. Developing-country research often takes place in communities where people live and work in close proximity. People who don't participate in studies hear stories about research from neighbors and relatives enrolled in trials. Some community members have participated in previous studies in the area, and some will be asked to join future investigations. For these individuals, human research is not a one-time event; it is an ongoing activity that touches their own lives and those of others in the community.[6]

In developing-country research, community residents are often members of the research team too. Some are hired to serve as fieldworkers performing the everyday tasks that research requires. Local health workers and "village reporters" are enlisted to provide study information and help with recruitment and care of study participants. These research staff members usually live among or even with study participants and their families.[7] Such arrangements foster unusually close relationships between research staff and participants, "conflat[ing] the categories of observer and observed."[8] They also affect expectations of privacy and confidentiality.

As I discussed in previous chapters, community engagement is a strategy that gives prospective and actual research subjects a voice in research. Community engagement has a long history in the developing world. As early as the 1970s, researchers in developing countries began collaborating with local communities to plan and carry out projects.[9] In the years since then, social scientists and others engaged in such collaborations have collected a wealth of information about how people in host communities think about research. Empirical research examining community perceptions has flourished.

Years of investigations of this kind have produced a rich literature, one that includes extensive information about the perspectives of experienced research participants and people close to them. In turn, social scientists have developed a relatively sophisticated understanding of how experienced subjects and other community members think about research. Their findings have led some social scientists to criticize standard accounts of ethics for global research.

According to the critics, standard ethics accounts often reflect simplistic assumptions about how people in developing countries think about research.[10] Critics also point out that "differences in cultural understandings mean that internationally 'agreed' ethical principles can be interpreted in varied and unexpected ways."[11] They contend as well that standard ethics accounts fail to consider how personal relationships affect study ethics.

Social scientists describing these problems believe that ethicists have been insufficiently attentive to empirical data describing local perspectives on research. Two social scientists with years of experience observing health studies in Africa put it this way:

> Ethics debates tend to be dominated by the views of scientists and advocates from high-income settings, or by professionals from low-income countries who have had little opportunity to engage in the actual conduct of studies. The perceptions and priorities of the diverse communities who are the subjects of research, of the local researchers and research assistants who are primarily responsible for implementing "ethically appropriate" practices, and of the health workers, managers and policy makers who are so often expected to put research findings into practice, are therefore rarely heard.[12]

To correct the situation, social scientists urge ethicists to develop an "embedded ethics" that takes into account the views of research participants and others who live in the community.[13] Developing an embedded ethics will require ethicists to look more closely at "what happens when one person responds to the other in open-ended, face-to-face relations that occur within the field, in everyday research."[14]

In the rest of this chapter, I show how embedded ethics can enrich the standard understanding of research ethics. I give examples of what research participants and others living in developing countries say about the benefits and burdens of research participation, the consent process, and the role research plays in their communities. I also report on how relationships among people involved in trials affect research ethics.

The empirical findings on developing-country research complicate and challenge accepted ethical principles, revealing how ethics plays out in real-world settings. The findings are graphic and poignant as well. Like other material in this book, accounts from participants in developing-country research and those close to them bring to light otherwise neglected features of human research.

The material in this chapter also highlights the global disparities that can shape how research is conducted. Interviews and discussions with people in developing-country communities reveal resourcefulness and resilience but also need and vulnerability. Personal accounts illuminate and emphasize the social justice concerns that arise in developing-country research.

THE BROAD ETHICAL FRAMEWORK FOR DEVELOPING-COUNTRY RESEARCH

Clinical trials in developing countries should meet general ethical standards for human research. This means that researchers should treat study participants with respect. People living in low-income countries should understand what research participation involves before making their choices about it, and they should not feel unduly pressured to sign up for studies. As in other research settings, people should be free to decide for themselves whether to join trials.

Study teams in developing countries face a variety of challenges in promoting informed and voluntary consent. Written consent forms are of limited use in places where few people are able to read. People unfamiliar with science and medicine need trial explanations they can understand. Decisions by people who live on very little can be influenced by the prospect of receiving small amounts of money or other forms of study compensation. Community members may look to leaders and representatives for guidance on whether to be involved in studies. Women may seek their husbands' permission before consenting to study participation.

Research in developing countries should also present an acceptable balance of benefits and burdens. Risks and burdens must be minimized, and benefits must be sufficient to justify negative impacts of a study. Applying this principle requires close examination of the local context in which studies occur, for research participation can involve distinct burdens and benefits for people in low-income countries.

Local conditions affect research burdens. In small communities, privacy can be hard to maintain. In some communities, people diagnosed with communicable diseases like HIV and tuberculosis (TB) face stigma and discrimination. If their disease status becomes known to the wider community, they could lose jobs, homes, and personal relationships. Allowing research staff into one's home can also trigger suspicion, envy, or resentment in others. The demands that research puts on local health workers and facilities can reduce community members' access to customary medical care.[15]

At the same time, research in developing countries can bring with it an array of otherwise unavailable benefits. Subjects can receive medication and other help with health problems that normally go unattended. Their families can get healthcare too. Research teams can also provide much-needed money, food, and other necessities of everyday life.[16]

The primary benefit of research is knowledge, of course. But there are serious questions about who benefits from the knowledge generated through research in low-income countries. Too often, researchers from wealthy countries come to low-income countries to conduct studies whose main benefits go to people in wealthy countries. Research subjects in poor countries often don't have access to the health improvements they helped produce. This is an unfair and unjust distribution of research burdens and benefits.[17]

Ethics and policy experts have proposed various requirements aimed at preventing this kind of research exploitation. According to one such requirement, any drug or other intervention found to benefit study subjects should be made "reasonably available" to subjects after the study is over. Some observers say that beneficial study interventions should also be supplied to other individuals living in the same community or country.[18]

But because single studies rarely point to a drug or other intervention's being clearly beneficial, the reasonable-availability requirement fails to ensure that subjects and their communities will benefit from research. The "fair benefits" requirement is meant to address this shortcoming. According to the fair-benefits requirement, all studies must provide some benefits to participants and their communities. Research teams must make contributions that are valuable to the host community, such as training health workers and establishing new clinics. Contributions like these can offer clear and long-lasting benefits to research participants and to the communities that hosted the researchers.[19] A related approach called "relief of oppression" urges researchers to contribute benefits that relieve background conditions of injustice in host communities.[20]

Other research requirements seek to ensure fair distributions of benefits versus burdens by directing researchers to address the most serious health needs of host countries or communities. This approach supports an increased research focus on problems like TB, HIV, malaria, and morbidity and mortality of mothers and children in sub-Saharan Africa.[21]

Community engagement is another ethical requirement for developing-country research. Ethicists and policymakers call for collaboration and partnership when research sponsored by wealthy countries is conducted in low-income countries.[22] Every facet of research, from setting research priorities to designing, conducting, and reviewing the ethics of individual studies, should involve people living in the host community. Host community researchers, clinicians, leaders, and local residents all have a part in promoting ethical research.

Meeting these and other ethical requirements requires close attention to the views of people living in the communities where research is conducted. Experienced research participants should be part of this focus. As the empirical literature reveals, people who participate in developing-country research can supply information relevant to evaluating participant benefits and burdens, consent procedures, study participation incentives, community benefits, and community engagement.

PARTICIPANT BENEFITS

People in developing countries enroll in research for a variety of reasons. Like research subjects in developed countries, people in developing countries sometimes enroll as a way to obtain potential treatment for the health problem under study. Through participating in research, people can gain access to potential preventive measures like vaccines as well.[23]

People in developing countries also enroll in research to obtain what is known as "ancillary care." This is "medical care that the research subjects need but that is not required to make a study scientifically valid, to ensure a study's safety, or to redress research injuries."[24] Ancillary care can be a huge motivator for subjects in developing countries. Joining a study allows some people to receive care they wouldn't otherwise get. It can allow subjects to bypass overcrowded health clinics with long waiting lines. Study participation can open the door to healthcare for family members too.[25]

People in developing countries say they receive psychological benefits from research participation as well. Some use words like "hospitality" to describe their research experience.[26] Fieldworkers and other research staff members in the community can become like family and friends to study subjects.[27] Participants in an HIV trial in Kenya "talked about 'feeling nice' when visited" by research staff, and some even "evoked 'love' to describe their special bond."[28] A study subject in the Philippines told interviewers: "[T]he women who were employed to interview us . . . treated us like sisters. Sometimes they would get tears when we were giving our responses."[29]

Monetary and in-kind compensation are additional benefits that attract people to research participation. Besides cash payments and reimbursement of expenses, volunteers can receive food, mosquito nets, and other useful goods. These rewards can be quite appealing. For example, study participants in Malawi said that "when they took part in research, they earned money without having worked or labored for it."[30] One participant said that some people who initially refused to join studies would change their minds "when they saw that others had been given presents."[31]

But not everyone in developing countries sees this sort of compensation as appropriate. In South Africa, for example, a group of potential and actual research participants told interviewers that "it was not right to want something in return for helping their own communities."[32] One person thought it would be unwise to take money in exchange for assuming research risks. "I won't go for money. Money can't do anything. If my health is suffered, then what?" she asked. "I am going to eat that money?"[33] These individuals said that improving health in their communities was the main reason to volunteer.

Many subjects in developing countries agree that research produces new knowledge and that this new knowledge can be beneficial. As one put it, "From the findings the doctors will gain more knowledge to treat people in the future so that they will benefit even more than us."[34] Yet subjects sometimes question whether research yields valuable knowledge. For example, female sex workers in the Philippines told interviewers that their extensive past research participation had failed to produce improvements in their lives. One said that what they really needed was "help for some of us to go back to school, improve how to speak English so that we can apply to a call center, or have trainings about cooking, dressmaking or other livelihoods that would help us gain opportunities to work in another country."[35]

PARTICIPANT RISKS AND BURDENS

Besides the usual physical risks that accompany trial participation, people in developing countries face risks and burdens related to their social and cultural situations. As I noted earlier, privacy and confidentiality are major concerns in certain areas. Clinic visits and interactions with research staff can reveal a subject's disease status or other stigmatizing information to relatives and neighbors. Study subjects also wonder whether the research staff can be trusted to keep information confidential.

Social scientists report many examples of these concerns. A Ghanaian TB study participant told interviewers: "Scientific research is risky in many ways. First thing is that I do not know you well and secondly I do not know exactly where they will be taking the material they collect so that is a risk. It is possible that someone will know that I have this disease and blame me for spreading it in the neighborhood so it is risky."[36] Female sex workers participating in HIV studies in India worried about privacy too. Some complained that study staff members were "conducting interviews at the hotspots under the trees in front of others."[37] One women was upset because someone on the staff gave participants their HIV test results in groups rather than individually.

Concerns like these are not unfounded, for research participants in developing countries can suffer severe consequences if others learn of their disease status. For example, female sex workers in the Philippines worried about being arrested and losing their jobs if their HIV survey responses were disclosed to others.[38] Some women in a Kenyan HIV study went to great lengths to keep their participation secret from their husbands, hiding medication and study documents and running away when staff visited their homes. They weren't always successful, however, and the discovery of a wife's HIV diagnosis led some husbands to end the relationship. Some of the women then became homeless, because they couldn't afford to rent living spaces of their own.[39]

Research-related rumors can also be disturbing to subjects and their families. In one Kenyan community, for example, the involvement of male fieldworkers in a malaria vaccine trial triggered rumors of romantic relationships with mothers of children enrolled in the trial. People also suspected that researchers had a hidden agenda. There were rumors that researchers would secretly test blood samples for HIV, sell samples for profit, give them to devil worshippers, or use them to provide transfusions to others. As the trial proceeded without incident, participants became less troubled by the rumors but still worried that "their journey with the research team" could go awry. As one mother commented, "In a traffic accident, the driver dies with the passengers."[40]

Another common concern is that researchers will abandon the people who helped them with their studies. Kenyans enrolled in the malaria vaccine trial feared that researchers would leave them with nothing. They wanted a public statement or gift in appreciation for the efforts they had made. They also wanted researchers to leave something valuable behind, such as drugs, free vaccines, and a clinician to care for trial participants, "so the PI does not benefit alone" and "those that did not consent for the study . . . feel bad."[41] If trial benefits were to end abruptly, one parent said, "We'll become a laughing stock."[42]

Like subjects in developed countries, subjects in developing countries want research teams to treat them with courtesy, sensitivity, and respect. But again like subjects elsewhere, subjects in developing countries don't always receive such treatment. Study participants in developing

countries describe dealing with long waits, rushed interviews, and insensitive or untrained staff.[43] To sex workers in
India, having separate bathrooms for staff and subjects was
a sign that staff "looked down on us."[44] These women also
reported truly outrageous behavior by a few male researchers, including an investigator "who returned as a client with
friends after the research was completed."[45]

Subjects are sometimes disturbed by study procedures
too. For example, sex workers in India and the Philippines
were offended by some of the questions survey researchers
asked them, such as "if I have sex when I'm drunk, do I use
condoms, how many partners do I have." Subjects felt these
questions were intrusive. "No one is comfortable answering
these questions," one said.[46]

Participants have other kinds of complaints about
their past research experiences. A female sex worker in the
Philippines said, "since I started to work in this kind of industry and participated in so many different research studies, I don't feel and see the appropriate programs for us . . .
because I'm still here!"[47] Two South Africans who had previously participated in research said they would not do so
again, because, as one put it, "In those old days they would
just come and take blood and . . . never explain to us what
they are doing."[48]

These empirical data reveal the value of consulting experienced subjects about potential benefits and harms of a
proposed study. Experienced subjects know about benefits
and harms that might otherwise remain unrecognized or
underappreciated. They reveal the price participants can pay
when the research staff fail to protect their privacy as well
as the disrespectful treatment that can come from research
teams preoccupied with their own agendas. Research teams

need information from experienced subjects to design and conduct studies that present a defensible balance of risks and benefits to participants.

POST-TRIAL BENEFITS TO PARTICIPANTS AND COMMUNITIES

As I said earlier, there is a growing consensus that research conducted in developing countries should benefit those countries. In surveys and interviews, social scientists have asked experienced subjects and others in host communities what those benefits ought to be. In many cases, subjects and other community residents have similar ideas on this topic. In some cases, however, people with experience as research subjects express views that differ from those of people lacking this experience.

One team found both commonalities and differences among the Ugandan community leaders, residents, and participants in infectious disease trials they surveyed. The survey asked people in these groups about the benefits that researchers conducting an HIV vaccine trial should provide to the community. Nearly half of all survey respondents thought that researchers should provide healthcare services as post-trial benefits. Other popular choices were clinics, clean water, money, and the trial vaccine (if it proved to be effective). Eighty percent of all respondents opposed limiting post-trial benefits to vaccine trial participants. Instead, they thought that benefits should go to everyone in the local community. Many also thought that benefits other than the vaccine were most important, because of the "tangible, pressing needs in their community."[49]

Among the differences the survey team found in how experienced subjects and other groups thought about research was that "active research participants were less likely than others to say that researchers should compensate participants, but more likely to say that money should be provided to the community."[50] Respondents from all groups thought that people who had participated in research should have a leading role in evaluating community benefits. When asked who should decide on post-trial benefits, 31 percent of those surveyed preferred community leaders. But 22 percent preferred experienced research participants as the decision makers.

Other surveys on post-trial benefits have addressed the reasonable-availability question. A Brazilian survey asked experienced research participants, research sponsors, study investigators, and ethics committee chairs who should receive beneficial study medication or equivalent therapy after a trial is completed. There were striking differences in how the groups responded. Sixty percent of experienced research participants thought that all patients, both trial participants and others, should get medication; support for this position was lower in the other groups. Experienced participants were also more likely than other groups to believe that medication should be free and that trial participants should receive medication for the rest of their lives.[51]

Another reasonable-availability survey showed similar divisions. Experienced research participants, investigators, and ethics committee chairs in eleven countries (several of which were developing countries) responded to this survey. Eighty-three percent of the experienced participants believed that "every HIV-infected person should receive the study drug if beneficial." In contrast, just 42 percent of investigators and 29 percent of the ethics committee chairs took this position.[52]

Data from surveys like these suggest that experienced subjects should be part of the discussion of post-trial benefits. One can argue that experienced participants earn a place in such decision-making through their personal contributions to studies. In the Ugandan survey, quite a few respondents thought that participants were the group most qualified to make decisions about post-trial benefits. And participants' survey responses show that they are deeply invested in the well-being of their wider communities.

UNDERSTANDING AND VOLUNTARINESS IN STUDY DECISIONS

Relatively low literacy rates, the pressures of poverty, and other features of life in developing countries raise concerns about the quality of participants' decisions to enroll in research. Empirical evidence suggests that these concerns are often valid. Yet the evidence does not show that research decisions are inevitably deficient in developing countries. As one review of research on informed consent stated, to assume that "informed consent is worse in developing countries than in developed countries is a simplification of a complex picture."[53]

That review, which covered forty-seven studies that evaluated subject understanding of consent in developed and developing countries, describes numerous complexities. According to the review team, the studies as a whole "do not support a categorical difference between the quality of consent from individuals in developed countries and the quality of consent from individuals in developing countries."[54] Subjects in both developed and developing countries generally understood why trials were being done and what they would involve. On the other hand, subjects in both developed and developing countries lacked a good understanding of research methods like randomization and the use of placebo-control groups.

Individual consent is important to many people in developing countries. For example, although members of a Kenyan community recognized difficulties in informing people about research, most thought that this was a necessary task. As one woman put it: "If I agree they can go ahead but if they do it without asking me then they're in the wrong. We have to understand each other before extra blood is taken."[55]

The best methods for promoting informed decisions are a matter of debate among people living in developing countries. In interviews and focus groups in Ghana, for example, experienced subjects and parents of children in research expressed a variety of opinions on the value of written consent forms. Some individuals who couldn't read preferred a verbal process, but others wanted both verbal and written information, noting that they could have someone else read the written form to them. Some liked having the form to take home as a reminder even though they couldn't read it. Some also believed that having this record might help them secure research benefits in the future.[56]

Although individual informed consent is important to people in developing countries, the consent of others can be important to them as well. One popular view is that members of the broader community should have an opportunity to weigh in on proposed trials: before approaching individuals about possible trial participation, researchers should explain their studies to leaders and other community representatives and obtain their permission to proceed. Although people define community consent in different ways, some form of initial community consent has been endorsed by potential and actual research participants in many developing countries.[57]

Few people see community consent as a substitute for individual consent, however. For example, in a Kenyan community discussion, one woman said: "It is important for the fieldworkers to get permission from the chief to move around the area, but the chief cannot decide for my child. No way!"[58] Leaders said they saw themselves as information sources for individuals in the community rather than as decision makers for those individuals. In northern Ghana, chiefs and elders also felt their authority was limited. Indeed, even when they were unhappy with an investigator's performance they did not intervene in the research.[59]

Consultation with relatives and friends can also be important to people considering research participation. Seventy-eight percent of Nigerian participants in a genetic study said that they had talked with family members or friends before joining the study. Thirty-nine percent of them had asked a spouse or other relative for permission to enroll, with half of the women seeking permission from their husbands.[60] In a rural community in Ghana, all of the women in focus groups said that they consulted their husbands before participating in research, with some requiring their husbands' permission and others making the choice

themselves.[61] In small group discussions, most members
of a Kenyan community said that the man of a household
should make the decision about a child's research participation and that children should not be involved in that
choice.[62]

Trust plays a big role in decisions to participate in research too. People living in communities that have established research centers sometimes assume that any project from the center will be beneficial.[63] Examples of this
thinking come from vaccine trial participants in Kenya.
In group discussions, it became evident that for some participants, the choice to enroll "had less to do with any of
the study details ... than with previous encounters with,
and confidence in, the research centre."[64] One woman described how her baby's earlier involvement in an epilepsy
study motivated her own decision to join the vaccine
trial: "[T]he baby took drugs, her condition got better and
now she's OK. So now, when this [research center] activity
about malaria came, I saw no problem. I hurriedly went
and underwent their processes."[65]

A related way of thinking emerged in other interviews
with members of a Kenyan community, including parents
whose children had been in trials. Community members
generally described the area's research center as an operation that provided healthcare, "despite years of staff regu-
larly visiting and explaining their work."[66] According to the
interview team, people commonly believed that research
activities were designed to benefit participants—the belief
known as the therapeutic misconception (see chapter 3).
When discussing study procedures that were hard to fit into
the category of therapy, local residents came up with other
reasons for the procedures. For example, they thought that

extra blood samples would be used to give transfusions to other patients.

Some projects in developing countries present a different picture, however. For example, interviews with TB study participants in Ghana found a relatively high level of understanding among participants. Most of the group were aware of the knowledge-gathering objective of research, with 70 percent responding that advancing knowledge was a major benefit of research. One participant in the group offered this apt description: "[R]esearch is like doing criminal investigative work. You are looking for sources and causes of things, in this particular case, the causes of diseases."[67]

The interviews in Ghana also highlight an important aspect of evaluating participant understanding in developing countries. The study procedures in the Ghanaian research had no chance of directly benefiting the participants. But participants saw the trial as potentially beneficial, for it offered them TB education and treatment for active TB. Because these were actual ancillary-care benefits that the study team provided, the participants' belief that the trial was beneficial was accurate.

Social scientists point out that research teams in developing countries usually provide ancillary-care benefits to research participants. In this situation, participants who see healthcare as a research benefit are not wrong. As one team observed, "To render this experience as a 'therapeutic misconception' fails to acknowledge the realities of the local situation."[68] Consistent with this view, another team concluded that when trial participants in Malawi said they joined studies to get better medical treatment, they were making an informed and rational choice rather than one that reflected a misunderstanding of the facts.[69]

Yet providing ancillary-care benefits also has a downside, for it can make participants less attentive to the extra burdens that research imposes. Researchers who provide ancillary care to participants may have a harder time explaining risks associated with the knowledge-seeking elements of their studies. As a team in Kenya observed, "meeting one ethical requirement (for example ensuring that potential participants are given basic health care) can compromise another (for example ensuring that potential participants can distinguish clinical research from practice and thereby make an informed decision)."[70]

Another concern is that the prospect of receiving ancillary care will induce people in developing countries to enroll in research. Ancillary-care benefits are one of several factors that can compromise the voluntariness of a person's research choices. Yet empirical data reveal that the "subjective experiences of social and economic constraints on voluntariness are neither uniform nor necessarily predictable."[71]

Empirical studies show that the desire to obtain potential therapies, ancillary care, and other benefits that come with study participation can strongly motivate people in developing countries to enroll in research. But these motivations don't necessarily compromise the voluntariness of their choices. For example, rural Kenyan parents whose children participated in a malaria vaccine study said that they "joined of their own free will knowing that they could withdraw whenever they wished."[72] Similarly, people in Malawi who enrolled in research to secure healthcare and other ancillary benefits said that they did not feel forced to enroll. One participant said: "I wanted better medical help. They told me that I was free to opt out if I wanted to. But

I accepted because I wanted to receive better drugs and get well quickly."[73] Community members in Kenya were more concerned about the unfairness of giving participants too few benefits than about the risk that too many benefits would compromise individual free choice.[74]

This is not to suggest that people in developing countries always feel free to refuse research. For example, some sex workers in the Philippines felt pressure from the government to participate in HIV survey research.[75] The group that reviewed forty-seven studies on research decision making concluded that "a disquieting number of participants, and more in developing country trials than in developed country trials, do not know or do not believe that they can refuse to participate or can withdraw from research."[76] The review team suggested that cultural beliefs, fear of being denied healthcare, or respect for authority figures could explain this situation.

People who enroll in research because they feel pressure to do so sometimes become "silent refusers." Silent refusers miss or postpone scheduled appointments, give "one-word answers [or] silence in response to questions," or ask workers to discuss study matters with other relatives.[77] Silent refusal is adopted by people who either are intimidated by research workers or hope to obtain study benefits without undergoing all of the study procedures.

In sum, empirical data on research decision making present a mixed picture. Although some participants understand and freely consent to research, others do not. Addressing the barriers to informed and voluntary choice requires close attention to the social conditions and power relationships in particular communities. The views of experienced participants should be part of the examination.

ETHICS AND COMMUNITY
ENGAGEMENT

Groups addressing the ethics of global research encourage researchers to create partnerships with local communities.[78] Consistent with this advice, research teams in developing countries often include local residents and other individuals who live in the country where the research takes place. When research staff members live among and with participants, personal relationships and day-to-day interactions "form the fabric in which the dialogue, information sharing and negotiations that are central to ethical practice take place."[79] Yet the formal ethical principles governing developing-country research fail to address the ethics of these relationships and interactions. Besides general ethical principles and ethics review committees, developing-country research requires an ethics of engagement.[80]

As I noted earlier, community engagement is a long-standing and widespread practice in developing-country research. A major goal of engagement is to make research more ethical. Engagement is intended to create an "opportunity for research participants and affected communities to voice their concerns, and for researchers to acknowledge them and respond constructively."[81] But meaningful community engagement requires strong commitment and extensive local knowledge.

Anthropologists, sociologists, and others examining developing-country research are well aware of on-the-ground challenges to making community engagement work. They are also aware of the ethical issues that can arise when research teams, community members, and study participants interact. Through interviews, focus groups, and other empirical investigations, they have detected an array of issues that warrant further ethical examination.

The Embedded Research Staff

The success of trials in developing countries is often attributed to the presence of an embedded research staff. For example, local fieldworkers were largely responsible for carrying out a successful malaria vaccine trial in the Gambia. A review team found that participants had very positive views of the trial, largely because they valued the local fieldworkers' contributions. Participants liked the convenience of local research appointments as well as the easily accessible ancillary healthcare the fieldworkers provided. In turn, participants were highly cooperative with trial requirements, including follow-up measures. Participants saw themselves and the fieldworkers as members of a "trial family" rather than as two separate groups with different interests and agendas.[82]

Participants in a respiratory virus study in Kenya also had favorable responses to the embedded research staff. In that study, close interactions between participants and fieldworkers in places like markets were opportunities to become acquainted and talk about study concerns. Nearly all of the households asked to join the study agreed to do so, and only a few failed to complete it. The relationships between participants and fieldworkers were central to the trial's success.[83]

An embedded research staff can also enhance the benefits that research projects provide to developing-country communities. When local staff members receive training in healthcare delivery and disease control measures, they can continue their health work after research projects are complete. If done effectively and given adequate financial support, this knowledge transfer leaves a community with a better health infrastructure than it had before the research began, increasing the project's social value.[84]

Yet the close encounters that can be so beneficial are not problem-free. The involvement of local community health workers in a Kenyan vaccine trial raised ethical concerns about worker-participant interactions. In interviews, parents complained that some workers overemphasized study benefits and tried to pressure them to enroll their children. A father who decided not to enroll his child said of one worker: "She tried to explain more to me and she thought that I had not understood about the study. Therefore, she came to me again and explained again very well and I absolutely understood her but then the decision is, I had already decided."[85]

Other investigations describe similar issues related to "the potentially manipulative power of intimacy."[86] In some studies in Kenya, fieldworkers reportedly "hyped up" potential study benefits and tried to convince people to enroll. When participants were considering withdrawing from studies, fieldworkers tried to change their minds.[87] Households that developed close relationships with certain fieldworkers failed to cooperate with new staff members brought in to handle increasing study demands.[88]

Dealing with households like these is just one of the ethical challenges local fieldworkers can face. Research participants have many needs, and fieldworkers come face to face with those needs. This happened in the Kenyan respiratory virus study described earlier. As the study participants and fieldworkers grew closer, "[r]equests by participants for benefits and gifts beyond those officially provided by the study, such as for food items, cell phone airtime, and baby clothes, became increasingly common."[89] Fieldworkers in another African vaccine trial with no clear provisions governing ancillary medical care faced participants and families in need of such care. Local research staff struggled to do what they could with few resources. In this situation, "the key ethical question for [fieldworkers] and the villagers was not whether they provided the best care at all times to those entitled, but that they made an effort when faced with suffering."[90]

Friendships between research workers and participants give rise to additional issues. These friendships are threatened when participants don't cooperate with study requirements. Participants may become overly casual with workers, failing to respect professional boundaries and threatening workers' professional reputations.[91] Workers may have to decide whether deception is justified to protect study participants from potentially violent husbands and other relatives.[92]

Community Representatives

Community engagement involves more than appointing local residents to a research staff. Through public meetings and other forms of publicity, research teams supply communities with project information. Local residents are designated to represent communities through service on community advisory boards or participation in gatherings at which proposed studies are described. As I mentioned earlier, sometimes a form of community consent is part of the engagement process.

Choosing people to represent a community is an important part of engagement. The choice of representatives partly depends on how the relevant community is defined—by location, interests, or perspectives. Representatives are chosen by researchers or through a community selection process.[93] Community leaders and healthcare workers are often named as representatives. Individuals are also chosen to represent specific groups or to supply "typical community views."[94]

The choice of representatives has ethical implications. What gives a person authority to speak on behalf of a particular group? Are some selection methods more legitimate than others? Is the selection process open to women and members of other traditionally excluded groups? What sort of information gathering enables a person to speak on behalf of a community group?[95]

Groups and individuals addressing the ethics of community engagement point to additional issues. People involved in community engagement may seek to manipulate the process to serve their own ends. Researchers and others may be hostile to engagement, seeking to defeat it in overt and covert ways. Vulnerable groups can be shut out when powerful people dominate engagement activities. Dealing with the inevitable differences of opinion among community representatives or between researchers and community representatives is another engagement challenge.[96]

The literature on community engagement in developing countries is thoughtful and enlightening, exposing many issues that merit further examination. There is one major deficiency in the literature, however. Although writers recognize the ethical dimensions of engagement, they have yet to recognize the distinct value that experienced study participants can bring to community engagement activities. Community members on the research staff and representatives of the general community know something about the participant experience, but actual participants know more about it. The representation of experienced subjects should be explicitly recognized as an essential element of good community engagement.

EXPANDING EMBEDDED ETHICS

Embedded ethics widens the territory for ethical reflection on developing-country research. It's not enough for studies to conform to the general ethical principles that have so far been the focus in global-research ethics. A look at the real-life details of individual studies reveals the need for an ethics of person-to-person interactions. In the words of one experienced study team, "Ethical practice under the difficult conditions of overseas medical research can . . . only be generated through open-ended exploration of personal relations."[97]

Social scientists examining personal relations and interactions in the context of research offer strategies for making developing-country research more ethical. For example, explaining research concepts like randomization and double-blind designs using examples from agriculture or other activities of everyday life enhances understanding among low-literacy participants.[98] Giving people plenty of time to make research decisions allows them to consult relatives and friends whose opinions they respect.[99] Requiring research teams to train local health workers promotes fair benefits in global research.[100]

As the material described in this chapter reveals, however, generalizations about developing-country research are often inaccurate. Social scientists say that descriptions of "cultural differences between populations, or descriptions of community views as homogeneous, closed and static, mask a far more complex reality."[101] They point to "the centrality of context" in determining whether a study is ethical.[102] Taking context into account requires talking with the people most affected by a proposed study—the subjects, families, neighbors, and workers living in a study location.

Research ethicists should heed this call to delve into the details of developing-country research. The failure to look closely at real-world relationships and interactions generates an anemic research ethics. Principles and platitudes are of little use to research teams trying to develop effective community partnerships and conduct defensible studies in resource-poor areas.

The lessons of embedded ethics reach beyond the developing world. Researchers and ethicists in developed countries should pay more attention to the ways in which daily interactions and relationships affect research ethics. In this respect, the developing world has much to teach the developed world. Embedded ethics belongs in developed-country research too.

NOTES

1. Norimitsu Onishi and Sheri Fink, "Vaccines Face Same Mistrust That Fed Ebola," *New York Times*, March 13, 2015. Retrieved January 8, 2016, from http://www.nytimes.com/2015/03/14/world/africa/ebola-vaccine-researchers-fight-to-overcome-public-skepticism-in-west-africa.html.
2. Miriam Shuchman, "Ebola Vaccine Trial Faces Criticism," *Lancet* 385 (2015): 1933–34.
3. Onishi and Fink, "Vaccines Face Same Mistrust."

4. John-Arne Rottingen, "Ebola Vaccine Trial in Guinea," *Lancet* 385 (2015): 2459–60.

5. Stacy Carter, "Beware Dichotomies and Grand Abstractions: Attending to Particularity and Practice in Empirical Bioethics," *American Journal of Bioethics* 9, no. 6–7 (2009): 76–77.

6. P. Wenzel Geissler et al., "'He Is Now Like a Brother, I Can Even Give Him Some Blood'—Relational Ethics and Material Exchanges in a Malaria Vaccine 'Trial Community' in the Gambia," *Social Science and Medicine* 67 (2008): 696–707.

7. See Vibian Angwenyi et al., "Working with Community Health Workers as 'Volunteers' in a Vaccine Trial," *Developing World Bioethics* 13 (2013): 38–47; Tracey Chantler et al., "Ethical Challenges That Arise at the Community Interface of Health Research: Village Reporters' Experiences in Western Kenya," *Developing World Bioethics* 13 (2013): 30–37.

8. Geissler et al., "'He Is Now Like a Brother,'" 701.

9. Andrea Cornwell and Rachel Jewkes, "What Is Participatory Research?," *Social Science and Medicine* 41 (1995): 1667–76.

10. C. S. Molyneux et al., "'Even If They Ask You to Stand By a Tree All Day, You Will Have to Do It (Laughter) . . . !': Community Voices on the Notion and Practice of Informed Consent for Biomedical Research in Developing Countries," *Social Science and Medicine* 61 (2005): 443–54.

11. Bridget Pratt et al., "Perspectives from South and East Asia of Clinical and Research Ethics: A Literature Review," *Journal of Empirical Research on Human Research Ethics* 9, no. 2 (2014): 52–67, 53.

12. Sassy Molyneux and P. Wenzel Geissler, "Ethics and the Ethnography of Medical Research in Africa," *Social Science and Medicine* 67 (2008): 685–95, 688.

13. Ann Kelly et al., "'Like Sugar and Honey': The Embedded Ethics of a Larval Control Project in the Gambia," *Social Science and Medicine* 70 (2010): 1912–19, 1913.

14. Geissler et al., "'He Is Now Like a Brother,'" 700.

15. Nancy Kass et al., "Applying Ethical Principles to International Community-Based Research: A Case Study from the Consortium to Respond Effectively to the AIDS-TB Epidemic (CREATE)," *IRB: Ethics & Human Research* 36, no. 3

(2014): 1–8; Angwenyi et al., "Working with Community Health Workers."

16. See Maureen Njue et al., "Benefits in Cash or in Kind? A Community Consultation on Types of Benefits in Health Research on the Kenyan Coast," *PLoS One* 10, no. 5 (2015): e0127842.

17. Alex London, "Responsiveness to Host Community Needs," in *The Oxford Textbook of Clinical Research Ethics*, ed. Ezekiel Emanuel et al. (New York: Oxford University Press, 2008), 737–48.

18. See Participants in the 2001 Conference on Ethical Aspects of Research in Developing Countries, "Moral Standards for Research in Developing Countries: From 'Reasonable Availability' to 'Fair Benefits,'" *Hastings Center Report* 34, no. 3 (2004): 17–27.

19. Rafael Dal-Re et al., "Protections for Clinical Trials in Low and Middle Income Countries Need Strengthening, Not Weakening," *BMJ* 349 (2014): g4254; Ezekiel Emanuel, "Benefits to Host Countries," in *The Oxford Textbook of Clinical Research Ethics*, ed. Ezekiel Emanuel et al. (New York: Oxford University Press, 2008), 719–28.

20. James Lavery et al., "'Relief of Oppression': An Organizing Principle for Researchers' Obligations to Participants in Observational Studies in the Developing World," *BMC Public Health* 10 (2010): 384.

21. London, "Responsiveness"; Council for International Organizations of Medical Sciences, *International Ethical Guidelines for Biomedical Research Involving Human Subjects* (2002). Retrieved January 16, 2016, from http://www.cioms. ch/publications/layout_guide2002.pdf.

22. Participants in the 2006 Georgetown University Workshop on the Ancillary-Care Obligations of Medical Researchers Working in Developing Countries, "The Ancillary-Care Obligations of Medical Researchers Working in Developing Countries," *PLoS Medicine* 5, no. 5 (2008): e90; Ezekiel Emanuel et al., "What Makes Clinical Research in Developing Countries Ethical? The Benchmarks of Ethical Research," *Journal of Infectious Diseases* 189 (2004): 930–37.

23. Joseph Mfutso-Bengo, Lucinda Manda-Taylor and Francis Masiye, "Motivational Factors for Participation in Biomedical Research: Evidence from a Qualitative Study of Biomedical Research Participation in Blantyre District, Malawi," *Journal of Empirical Research on Human Research Ethics* 10, no. 1 (2015): 59–64; Christine Grady et al., "Research Benefits for Hypothetical HIV Vaccine Trials: The Views of Ugandans in the Rakai District," *IRB: Ethics & Human Research* 30, no. 2 (2008): 1–7.

24. Henry Richardson, *Moral Entanglements: The Ancillary-Care Obligations of Medical Researchers* (New York: Oxford University Press, 2012), 2–3.

25. Kelly et al., "'Like Sugar and Honey'"; Geissler et al., "'He Is Now Like a Brother.'"

26. Geissler et al., "'He Is Now Like a Brother,'" 701.

27. Elizabeth Reed et al., "Confidentiality, Privacy, and Respect: Experiences of Female Sex Workers Participating in HIV Research in Andhra Pradesh, India," *Journal of Empirical Research on Human Research Ethics* 9, no. 1 (2014): 19–28.

28. Philister Adhiambo Madiega et al., "'She's My Sister-in-Law, My Visitor, My Friend'—Challenges of Staff Identity in Home Follow-Up in an HIV Trial in Western Kenya," *Developing World Bioethics* 13 (2013): 21–29, 26.

29. Reed et al., "Confidentiality, Privacy, and Respect," 22.

30. Mfutso-Bengo, Manda-Taylor, and Masiye, "Motivational Factors for Participation," 61.

31. Ibid.

32. Olga Zvonareva et al., "Engaging Diverse Social and Cultural Worlds: Perspectives on Clinical Research Benefits in International Clinical Research from South African Communities," *Developing World Bioethics* 15 (2015): 8–17, 13.

33. Ibid.

34. John Appiah-Poku, Sam Newton, and Nancy Kass, "Participants' Perceptions of Research Benefits in an African Genetic Epidemiological Study," *Developing World Bioethics* 11 (2011): 128–35, 131.

35. Lianne Urada and Janie Simmons, "Social and Structural Constraints on Disclosure and Informed Consent for HIV Survey Research Involving Female Sex Workers and Their Bar

Managers in the Philippines," *Journal of Empirical Research on Human Research Ethics* 9, no. 1 (2014): 29–40, 36.

36. Appiah-Poku, Newton, and Kass, "Participants' Perceptions," 133.
37. Reed et al., "Confidentiality, Privacy, and Respect," 21.
38. Urada and Simmons, "Social and Structural Constraints."
39. Madiega et al., " 'She's My Sister-in-Law,' " 25.
40. Caroline Gikonyo et al., "Taking Social Relationships Seriously: Lessons Learned from the Informed Consent Practices of a Vaccine Trial on the Kenyan Coast," *Social Science and Medicine* 67 (2008): 708–20, 713.
41. Ibid., 715.
42. Ibid., 718.
43. Reed et al., "Confidentiality, Privacy, and Respect."
44. Ibid., 24.
45. Ibid., 23.
46. Urada and Simmons, "Social and Structural Constraints," 33.
47. Ibid., 35.
48. Zvonareva, "Engaging Diverse Social and Cultural Worlds," 14.
49. Ibid.
50. Grady et al., "Research Benefits," 5.
51. Sonia Dainesi and Moises Goldbaum, "Post-trial Access to Study Medication: A Brazilian E-survey with Major Stakeholders in Clinical Research," *Journal of Medical Ethics* 38 (2012): 757–62.
52. Christine Pace et al., "Post-trial Access to Tested Interventions: The Views of IRB/REC Chairs, Investigators, and Research Participants in a Multinational HIV/AIDS Study," *AIDS Research and Human Retroviruses* 9 (2006): 837–41.
53. Amulya Mandava et al., "The Quality of Informed Consent: Mapping the Landscape. A Review of Empirical Data from Developing and Developed Countries," *Journal of Medical Ethics* 38 (2012): 356–65, 361.
54. Ibid.
55. Molyneux et al., " 'Even If They Ask,' " 446.
56. Paulina Tindana, Nancy Kass, and Patricia Akweongo, "The Informed Consent Process in a Rural African Setting: A Case

Study of the Kassena-Nankana District of Northern Ghana," *IRB: Ethics & Human Research* 28, no. 3 (2008): 1–6.

57. See Rachel Vreeman et al., "A Qualitative Study Using Traditional Community Assemblies to Investigate Community Perspectives on Informed Consent and Research Participation in Western Kenya," *BMC Medical Ethics* 13, no. 23 (2012): 1–11.

58. Molyneux et al., "'Even If They Ask,'" 446.

59. Paulina Tindana et al., "Aligning Community Engagement with Traditional Authority Structures in Global Health Research: A Case Study from Northern Ghana," *American Journal of Public Health* 101 (2011): 1857–67.

60. Pauline Osamor and Nancy Kass, "Decision-Making and Motivation to Participate in Biomedical Research in Southwest Nigeria," *Developing World Bioethics* 12 (2012): 87–95.

61. Tindana, Kass, and Akweongo, "Informed Consent Process."

62. Molyneux et al., "'Even If They Ask,'" 446.

63. Tindana, Kass, and Akweongo, "Informed Consent Process."

64. Gikonyo et al., "Taking Social Relationships Seriously," 712.

65. Ibid.

66. C. S. Molyneux, N. Peshu, and K. Marsh, "Understanding of Informed Consent in a Low-Income Setting: Three Case Studies from the Kenyan Coast," *Social Science and Medicine* 59 (2004): 2547–59, 2550.

67. Appiah-Poku, Newton, and Kass, "Participants' Perceptions," 132.

68. Geissler et al., "'He Is Now Like a Brother,'" 699.

69. Mfutso-Bengo, Manda-Taylor, and Masiye, "Motivational Factors for Participation."

70. C. S. Molyneux, N. Peshu, and K. Marsh, "Trust and Informed Consent: Insights from Community Members on the Kenyan Coast," *Social Science and Medicine* 61 (2005): 1463–73, 1470.

71. Participants in the Community Engagement and Consent Workshop, Kilifi, Kenya, "Consent and Community Engagement in Diverse Research Contexts: Reviewing and Developing Research and Practice," *Journal of Empirical Research on Human Research Ethics* 8, no. 4 (2013): 1–18, 5.

72. Gikonyo et al., "Taking Social Relationships Seriously," 714.

73. Mfutso-Bengo, Manda-Taylor, and Masiye, "Motivational Factors for Participation," 61.

74. Maureen Njue et al., "What Are Fair Study Benefits in International Health Research? Consulting Community Members in Kenya," *PLoS ONE* 9, no. 12 (2014): 1–21.

75. Urada and Simmons, "Social and Structural Constraints."

76. Mandava et al., "Quality of Informed Consent," 363.

77. Participants in the Community Engagement and Consent Workshop, "Consent and Community Engagement," 5; Molyneux, Peshu, and Marsh, "Understanding of Informed Consent," 2555.

78. See, for example, Emanuel et al., "What Makes."

79. Dorcas Kamuya et al., "Evolving Friendships and Shifting Ethical Dilemmas: Fieldworkers' Experiences in a Short-Term Community Based Study in Kenya," *Developing World Bioethics* 13 (2013): 1–9, 9.

80. Katherine King et al., "Community Engagement and the Human Infrastructure of Global Health Research," *BMC Medical Ethics* 15, no. 84 (2014): 1–6.

81. Ibid., 1.

82. Geissler et al., " 'He Is Now Like a Brother,' " 701.

83. Kamuya et al., "Evolving Friendships."

84. Kelly et al., " 'Like Sugar and Honey.' "

85. Angwenyi et al., "Working with Community Health Workers," 43.

86. Geissler et al., " 'He Is Now Like a Brother,' " 703.

87. Molyneux, Peshu, and Marsh, "Understanding of Informed Consent," 2554.

88. Kamuya et al., "Evolving Friendships," 6.

89. Ibid., 5

90. Geissler et al., " 'He Is Now Like a Brother,' " 705. See also Lavery et al., "Relief of Oppression," which discusses ways to calibrate the benefits that researcher teams supply to participants.

91. Kamuya et al., " 'Evolving Friendships,' " 8.

92. Madiega et al., "She's My Sister-in-Law."

93. See Dorcas Kamuya et al., "Engaging Communities to Strengthen Research Ethics in Low-Income Settings: Selection and Perceptions of Members of a Network of Representatives in Coastal Kenya," *Developing World Bioethics* 13 (2013): 10–20.

94. Ibid., 13.
95. I discuss these and related issues in chapter 2 of *When Science Offers Salvation: Patient Advocacy and Research Ethics* (New York: Oxford University Press, 2001).
96. See participants in the Community Engagement and Consent Workshop, "Consent and Community Engagement."
97. Geisler et al., " 'He Is Now Like a Brother,' " 705.
98. Paul Mdebele et al., "Improved Understanding of Clinical Trial Procedures among Low Literacy Populations: An Intervention within a Microbicide Trial in Malawi," *BMC Medical Ethics* 13 (2012): 1.
99. Osamor and Kass, "Decision-Making and Motivation," 93.
100. Kelly et al., " 'Like Sugar and Honey.' "
101. Molyneux et al., " 'Even If They Ask,' " 452.
102. Participants in the Community Engagement and Consent Workshop, "Consent and Community Engagement," 10.

8

Research Subjects
as Literary Subjects

■□■

CREATIVE WRITERS OFFER A DISTINCTIVE perspective on human research. Novels, short stories, plays, and other fictional works give researchers and research ethicists an opportunity to better understand the experience of becoming a human subject. Creative writers view research through the lens of ordinary people, but they are unusually perceptive and gifted "ordinary" people. They portray research experiences in fresh and insightful ways, and research professionals can learn from them.

Writers of fiction choose research as a dramatic setting because it offers a fertile context for exploring broader themes. In fiction, human experimentation creates intimacies between subjects and researchers. Through their interactions, characters in stories about research cope with fundamental human challenges, like the search for self and meaningful relationships with others. They also confront aging, disability, and mortality. Abuse of power, personal integrity, and the value of human life are additional common themes.

Subjects are the stars of many fictional research stories. Subjects in these stories have rich internal lives, as well as personal concerns and objectives that may or may not overlap with those of the researchers. Some fictional research volunteers are on a quest to improve their lives. Others don't join studies with that goal, yet still gain wisdom through their research experiences. Fictional research subjects are usually admirable or, at minimum, sympathetic characters. Subjects are nearly always the underdogs, and writers lead you to root for them. Even misbehaving subjects tend to occupy the higher moral ground.

Creative writers are deeply concerned with ethics. They may not cite the Nuremberg Code or the Belmont Report, but they are influenced by the principles in those documents. For the most part, creative writers portray research oversight as something positive but easy to get around. Writers often create morally suspect scientist characters who dismiss ethical concerns and operate under the radar of oversight committees. Yet the scientists usually pay a price. Oversight may be weak and ineffective, but renegade researchers rarely get away with their unethical behavior.

In the fiction I describe, subjects tell their side of the story. Certainly much is imagined—this is fiction, after all. At the same time, it's clear that the writers have conducted their own research, tracking down information about real-world human studies and sometimes drawing on personal research experience.

Creative writers have fashioned many memorable research stories; this chapter describes only some of them. I consider novels, plays, and short stories that take place in a research context.[1] I focus on work that emphasizes the research subject's perspective, although researchers also play a big role in these stories.

I begin with the classic research story, *Frankenstein*. With incredible foresight, Mary Shelley introduced many themes that recur in later fictional work. I proceed to describe how these and other themes appear in modern literature. In fiction, troubled research subjects achieve enlightenment, powerless subjects become powerful, subjects and researchers are flawed human beings, research rules are violated, and scientific goals are called into question. Fiction exposes features of human experimentation that other forms of research discourse rarely acknowledge.

AN UNFORGETTABLE RESEARCH SUBJECT

Two hundred years ago, Mary Shelley invented the most notorious experimental subject—Victor Frankenstein's monster.[2] A substantial part of *Frankenstein* is written from the subject's point of view. Shelley gives her research subject a loud and passionate voice. She vividly describes the monster's horrible acts, leaving no doubt that he is evil. When we read his side of the story, however, we see that he wasn't always a monster.

The experimental subject in *Frankenstein* begins as an innocent, childlike figure in need of protection and guidance. But the scientist, Frankenstein, abandons the "hideous monster" he created. Left to fend for himself, the monster learns to survive. He learns to speak and read too. In his concealed shelter near a family's cottage, he watches and becomes attached to his neighbors. Through observing their behavior, he develops a moral sense and longs to be a part of a community.

But when he tries to connect with the family, he encounters only fear and rejection. This is what makes him a monster. He describes to Frankenstein the source of his malevolence: "Everywhere I see bliss, from which I alone am irrevocably excluded. I was benevolent and good; misery made me a fiend. Make me happy, and I shall again be virtuous" (pp. 81–82).

The monster also reminds Frankenstein of their special relationship: "I am thy creature, and I will be even mild and docile to my natural lord and king if thy will perform thy part, that which thou owest me." Then the monster makes a promise. If Frankenstein will make him a female companion, they will both go to "the wilds of South America" and live together without hurting anyone. He begs Frankenstein, "let me feel gratitude towards you for one benefit!" (p. 125).

Frankenstein initially rejects the deal. But after the monster pleads with him, he changes his mind. Indeed, he sees "some justice" in the monster's request. The monster had shown he was "a creature of fine sensations, and did I not as his maker owe him all the portion of happiness that it was in my power to bestow?" (p. 125).

Yet Frankenstein can't bring himself to honor the bargain. He worries about the harm that could come from creating a mate for the monster. The female might be "ten thousand times more malignant than her mate." And what if they have offspring? Frankenstein refuses to "inflict this curse upon everlasting generations" (p. 144). As the monster watches, Frankenstein destroys the "creature on whose future existence [the monster] depended for happiness" (p. 145).

Devastated by what he has seen, the monster follows as Frankenstein tries to escape; eventually he murders his creator. Unlike Frankenstein, the monster does not offer an excuse for this behavior. The book ends with the monster's vow to punish himself by ending his own life.

Although Frankenstein claims concern for society as the justification for abandoning his subject, fear and shame are the true basis of his actions. Shelley forces him, as well as her readers, to see the situation from the experimental subject's vantage point. As critic Harold Bloom writes, "the monster is at once more intellectual and more emotional than his maker." Indeed, Bloom concludes, the "greatest and most astonishing achievement of Mary Shelley's novel is that the monster is *more human* than his creator."[3] Shelley's greatest sympathy lies with the monster, and she guides readers to the same position.

In *Frankenstein*, Shelley succeeds in making the most alien of research subjects—a monster—into a sympathetic figure. Identification with the subject, as well as other themes in Shelley's novel, recurs in more recent research fiction. The inner life of the subject, a topic that standard research accounts ignore, takes center stage in many fictional works. Subjects are agents, with desires and interests they pursue. Researchers are confronted with the full impact of their actions, and at times they are punished for what they do. Below I describe how modern writers portray the experience of being a human subject.

PARTICIPATION AND ENLIGHTENMENT

In modern fiction, becoming a research subject is often part of a troubled character's search for relief from a distressing situation. Sometimes the troubles are internal. Don DeLillo tells this kind of story in his 1986 novel *White Noise*.[4] In the novel, Babette, the wife of protagonist Jack Gladney, participates in a secret study of "Dylar," a drug she hopes will cure her "condition"—an unrelenting fear of death.

Jack is a professor, head of the department of Hitler studies at a local college. Babette, his fourth wife, is a busy mother, adult education teacher, and volunteer. They live with four of their many children and stepchildren. Although Jack believes that he and Babette have no secrets from each other, he is wrong about that. Babette's eleven-year-old daughter Denise discovers that her mother is taking a mysterious pill called Dylar. Whenever Jack or Denise asks about the pills, Babette is evasive, changing the subject. The medical authorities that Denise and Jack consult have never heard of Dylar.

Eventually Jack confronts Babette and demands an explanation. She reveals her condition and describes her search for a remedy. She initially tried self-help, but that was unsuccessful. Then one day she noticed a tabloid advertisement seeking volunteers for "secret research" (p. 192).

The study was Babette's "last resort," her "last hope" (p. 194). She got in touch with the project manager, Mr. Gray (a pseudonym), who agreed to consider her for the study. Her results on the screening tests showed she was an ideal subject, "extra sensitive to the terror of death" (p. 197). But to Babette and Mr. Gray's dismay, the study was put on hold. Gray's superiors at the drug company decided that more preclinical research was needed to evaluate whether the drug was safe enough for human testing.

Babette was desperate and refused to accept that decision. So instead, she tells Jack, "Mr. Gray and I made a private arrangement. Forget the priests, the lawyers, the psychobiologists. We would conduct the experiments on our own. I would be cured of my condition, he would be acclaimed for a wonderful medical breakthrough" (p. 193). The deal wasn't quite so straightforward, though, for Mr. Gray made one other demand. To get the drug, Babette would have to offer him her body, as well as her mind.

Jack is furious when he hears about the sex. But Jack also wants to try Dylar, for he shares Babette's obsession with death. And in the past few weeks he has become even more obsessed than usual, because he was recently exposed to a toxic chemical that was accidently released in their town. As a result, he is "tentatively scheduled to die" (p. 202). Babette won't help Jack get the drug, however, because taking Dylar was a mistake—it didn't work. But Jack no longer trusts his wife and thinks she is lying about that.

Jack goes to the motel where Mr. Gray lives, intending to shoot him and take his Dylar. He follows through on the first part of his plan, then regrets what he has done. Instead of taking the Dylar, he puts the wounded Gray in his car and drives around looking for a hospital. He finds a Roman Catholic clinic, where nuns care for Mr. Gray.

Jack and one of the nuns have a conversation about heaven and the afterlife. She tells him that she and the other nuns pretend to believe in these things, because other people need them to. Jack realizes that he is one of those people. He is moved by religious rituals even though he doesn't subscribe to them. He calms down and goes home to Babette and his children, surrendering to the uncertainties and absurdities of late twentieth-century American life.

In *White Noise*, research participation is part of a journey to enlightenment. Babette and Jack discover that science offers no remedy for their fear of death. Their only real, albeit imperfect, solace can come from each other, their children, and their community, united in the wait for mortality.

The lead character in David Gilbert's 2004 novel *The Normals*[5] is another individual who turns to research participation to cope with personal problems. Billy Schine is a Harvard graduate who needs to repay a $60,000 student loan. He isn't sure what to do with his life and is working temporary jobs while he searches for answers. Billy is also the only child of parents in declining health. His mother has dementia, and his father has asked Billy to help end their lives. On top of that, Billy hasn't been making his loan payments and is being hounded by a vicious debt collector.

Seeking a way out, Billy volunteers for a phase 1 study of an antipsychotic drug. The study will be conducted at the Animal Human Research Center (AHRC), a pharmaceutical company's residential test unit. By signing up for the study, Billy will not only earn $2,500; he will be out of his parents' and the debt collector's reach for a couple of weeks.

Volunteering does provide a certain level of escape. Billy finds "comfort here, in the routine, in the drift, in the purposeless purpose of the AHRC." During the trial, "he's sleepy and pleasantly removed from the process of survival. The sticky details of life are gone. All he has to do is swallow and bleed" (p. 210).

But Billy's move to the AHRC introduces a whole new set of problems. Life in the test unit resembles a soap opera. One of Billy's roommates is behaving more and more strangely, and Billy isn't sure what to do about it. Billy also develops a crush on one of his fellow subjects, but his feelings aren't reciprocated.

Then a doctor at the test facility tells Billy about a new research opportunity. The doctor is working on a method of temporarily freezing trauma victims. The goal is to extend the time that emergency room workers have to develop a treatment plan for their patients. Animal results have been encouraging, but drug regulators and company lawyers are blocking the doctor's effort to begin human trials.

Billy suggests that the doctor try the technique on him, in secret. From Billy's point of view, the study looks good. He sees his survival odds as "more than decent" (p. 295). He would be given $30,000, which would allow him to pay off a large part of his debt. And he would have an excuse for being absent on the occasion of his parents' planned death. Billy also hopes for something more from the experience. He tells the doctor: "Maybe a certain kind of focus would follow.... It might be the sort of depth experience I as a person need right now to settle things in my head a bit.... I just need something like this" (p. 252).

Billy's offer is accepted, but the test is a disaster and Billy almost dies. Nevertheless, his gamble pays off. Drug company officials fire the rogue researchers and pay Billy $250,000 for signing a nondisclosure agreement. Billy's money problems disappear. And much to Billy's surprise, his father shows up at the hospital where Billy is recuperating. It seems Billy's mother died naturally a few days before the couple's scheduled death. Billy is relieved that the plan didn't work out and that his father seems to have lost interest in killing himself. In ridiculous and unexpected ways, Billy's entry into the research world actually produced the solutions he was seeking.

Like Babette and Jack in *White Noise*, Billy Schine gains wisdom through his research encounter. His situation improves after he volunteers for research, but not in the way that he expected. He begins as an immature young man seeking to avoid his responsibilities. By the novel's end, he has grown up and can reconnect with the father he once sought to escape.

Some fictional characters join research in the hope that it will help with a different sort of threat, one posed by disease or disability. Although they don't necessarily expect the experience to confer wisdom or enlightenment, it does. In his 1966 novel *Flowers for Algernon*,[6] Daniel Keyes tells the story of one such character. At the beginning of the story, Charlie Gordon has an IQ of 68. He was born with a genetic condition that affected his mental abilities. Charlie is very aware of his disability and works hard to overcome it. He wants very much to "be smart." When offered an opportunity to participate in an experiment designed to increase intelligence, he eagerly volunteers.

The team conducting the experiment asks Charlie to write his own study progress report. *Flowers for Algernon* is that report. At first, Charlie's writing and spelling are primitive. At the same time, his innocence and good-heartedness shine through. We immediately sympathize with this unusual hero.

The experimental procedure seems to work, and Charlie's progress report becomes insightful and sophisticated. Eventually he is much more intelligent than anyone he knows. This is a mixed blessing. People Charlie formerly admired disappoint him. He turns against the researchers, refusing to cooperate with their plan to exhibit him to fellow scientists. In one of many outbursts, Charlie explains his position: "The problem, dear professor, is that you wanted someone who could be made intelligent but still be kept in a cage and displayed when necessary to reap the honors you seek. The hitch is that I'm a person" (p. 247).

As he becomes more aware of how the world works, Charlie gains a better understanding of his early life and family situation. He realizes that people mistreated him and becomes fiercely protective of his earlier self. What makes him most angry is that few people saw him as a person before he became intelligent. He now knows he was wrong to be ashamed of his previous disability.

The new and improved Charlie begins to investigate the science underlying his transformation. He discovers a flaw in the research team's thinking. Instead of producing a permanent change in intelligence, the technique will have only a temporary effect. Charlie anticipates his future as he watches the decline of Algernon, the mouse who was the initial subject in the intelligence experiment.

Soon Charlie's abilities are declining too. As he prepares for his new situation, he cuts off contact with the researchers. He tells a graduate student: "I'm through running the maze. I'm not a guinea pig any more." The student says that he understands, but Charlie disagrees. "You don't understand because it isn't happening to you" (p. 288).

Charlie goes to live in a home for mentally disabled people. His journal now exhibits the same primitive writing style it had at the start. In his final journal entry, Charlie vows to "keep trying to get smart" (p. 310). About his research experience he writes: "I bet Im the frist dumb persen in the world who found out something important for sience. I did something but I don't remembir what" (p. 311). Charlie closes his progress report by asking the researchers to leave flowers at the backyard grave where he buried Algernon.[7]

Through his research experience, Charlie discovers that what he once wanted so much is not as valuable as he thought. The experiment made him intelligent, but it deprived him of something more important, his genuine affection for other people. As he explains to the researchers, "When I was retarded I had lots of friends. Now I have no one" (p. 249). In his opinion, the experiment transformed him into "an arrogant, self-centered bastard" (p. 252). By the end of the novel, Charlie is his humble former self, someone we hope can once more care about others. The experimental procedure failed to help him, but he learned something important by becoming a research subject.

Vivian Bearing is another subject who learns what is truly important through her research experience. Vivian is the central character in Margaret Edson's 1995 play *Wit*.[8] Unlike Charlie, Vivian is a highly intelligent person when she becomes a research subject. A cancer patient facing her mortality, she has been enrolled in an experimental chemotherapy trial. Vivian was once a powerful and highly respected professor, but her situation changed when she was diagnosed with stage 4 metastatic ovarian cancer. Nature and the medical system have transformed her from a domineering authority figure to, as she sees it, a "simpering victim" with little control over her fate (p. 58).

Vivian struggles to maintain her dignity, but with little success. It doesn't help that Jason, the obtuse junior physician on the research team, is a former student of hers. He and his supervisor, Dr. Kelekian, are more concerned with their research objective—giving Vivian the maximum dose of the experimental regimen—than they are with their patient's welfare.

Vivian is quite aware of her role as a patient in an academic research center. She knows the game, and makes wry comments about it. At the same time, she shows us her suffering. For example, before Jason presents her case to his fellow trainees, Vivian sets the scene:

> In this dramatic structure you will see the most interesting aspects of my tenure as an in-patient receiving experimental chemotherapy for advanced metastatic ovarian cancer.
>
> But as I am a *scholar* before ... an impresario, I feel obliged to document what it is like here most of the time, between the dramatic climaxes. Between the spectacles.
>
> In truth, it is like this:
>
> You cannot imagine how time ... can be ... so still. It hangs. It weighs. And yet there is so little of it. It goes so slowly, and yet it is so scarce. (pp. 34–35)

Vivian plays along with the game because she can't admit to herself or the researchers that she is needy and dying. Her pride and fear make her vulnerable, and the physician-investigators take advantage of that. Only the nurse, Susie, treats her with compassion.

For better or worse, Vivian perseveres. Near the end of the play, she declares a research victory: she is still alive after eight doses of experimental chemotherapy. Having "broken the record," she has "become something of a celebrity." She suspects that Kelekian and Jason hope to become celebrities too, by publishing an article about her. Then she concedes that the "article will not be about *me*, it will be about my ovaries" (p. 53).

Vivian's true victory comes not from her valiant research performance, but from her acceptance of impending death. As the play concludes, she abandons her position as wry observer. This is not an abstract discussion, Vivian declares, "we are discussing my life and my death." It is "not the time for verbal swordplay, . . . for metaphysical conceit, for wit." Instead, it is "a time for simplicity" and "dare I say it, kindness" (p. 69).

Vivian is finally honest with herself and others. She tells Susie she realizes that Kelekian and Jason didn't expect the chemotherapy to cure her. She says she doesn't want to be resuscitated when her heart stops. No longer the stoic, she screams that she is in agonizing pain. She sees that that neither her own expertise nor the expertise of the researchers can save her. Opening herself to basic human connections is what helps her at the end. Once again, a research subject gains wisdom through her research experience.

VULNERABLE SUBJECTS: THE POWERLESS AS POWERFUL

In *Flowers for Algernon*, Charlie begins as a mentally disabled man easily manipulated by others. But he becomes, at least temporarily, a brilliant intellectual who discredits the scientific theory underlying his transformation. He also rejects the power games and shallow concerns that preoccupy the researchers and others who formerly looked down on him.

Flowers for Algernon is not the only story to portray a vulnerable subject who gets the better of researchers. In many stories, socially inferior subjects are revealed as morally superior to the researchers who mistreat them. Subjects are harmed and exploited in these stories, but they rise above it.

David Feldshuh's 1989 play *Miss Evers' Boys*[9] is one such story. The play is based on an actual research project, the US government–sponsored study of African American men with syphilis. From the 1930s to the 1970s, government researchers conducted the study in and around Tuskegee, Alabama. They withheld treatment from the men to learn about the natural course of the disease, and they used deception to secure the men's participation. The subjects were poor and uneducated, dependent on the research team for information and healthcare.

For dramatic purposes, the play takes liberties with the facts. The play has been criticized for suggesting that an African American research nurse, called "Miss Evers" in the play, was instrumental in convincing the men to cooperate with the study. Critics say that the real nurse, Eunice Rivers, simply behaved as nurses of that era were supposed to, doing what the white male researchers asked of her.[10]

What *Miss Evers' Boys* does well is to bring the research subjects to life. The men are neither silent nor docile. They initially object to the study, but are ordered to cooperate by the "white trash" owner of the land they farm. When the men meet Nurse Evers and the government researchers, they are skeptical and ask many questions about the study. The problem is that they don't receive truthful answers. As time goes by, Caleb, the most outspoken of the men, repeatedly expresses doubts about the project. When he learns that men in Birmingham are getting penicillin shots for syphilis, he gets one too, ignoring researchers' warnings that this would be risky.

The subjects in *Miss Evers' Boys* have rich lives and suffer heartbreaking losses as a result of their research involvement. In the early scenes, the men are skilled dancers, experts in their own right. But as the years pass without treatment, the physical impairments produced by syphilis destroy their hopes of becoming famous.

The play concludes in a waiting room outside a 1972 Senate hearing on the syphilis study. There, a subject named Willie forces the researchers to see his loss:

> You try to understand me. That penicillin would have made it so I could walk without pain and maybe even Jackspring [a dance move]. And they didn't give that to me in Birmingham because you pulled me out of that line so I could be a part of Miss Evers' Boys and Burial Society. So you all could do your watching while I wake up past midnight not feeling my legs or else feeling pain, burning pain, like a hot iron pressin' on my skin, 'til I shout, "Take this pain away. Lord, please, take this pain away." My body was my freedom. You hear me? MY BODY WAS MY FREEDOM. (p. 95)

Caleb is in the waiting room too. He is now Reverend Humphries, a respected member of the community. He tells the others that the newspapers are wrong to call the study worthless, for he actually did get "something useful out of all this" (p. 94). Years ago, as a token of appreciation, researchers had issued a certificate of participation to each study subject. Caleb announces that his certificate is now in the hands of the lawyers preparing a case against the government researchers.

Miss Evers' Boys graphically depicts the human costs of the Tuskegee syphilis study. Researchers took terrible advantage of the men, but Caleb and Willie have the last word. After the public learns about the study, the researchers will be widely condemned, and the men will receive compensation for their losses. In the end, it is the subjects who are the heroes of this research drama.

In his 2010 short story "Escape from Spiderhead,"[11] George Saunders features a different type of vulnerable subject. Jeff is a convicted criminal confined in a drug testing facility. Jeff and the other prisoners must participate in research—they have no real choice in the matter. Before each experiment, researchers ask subjects to "acknowledge" their agreement to proceed, but everyone knows this is a meaningless formality.

Jeff has been in therapy and is no longer the impulsive teenager whose violent actions led to his incarceration. He is also an unusually savvy and perceptive research subject, able to convey precise and objective reports on drug effects as he experiences them. Jeff understands scientific design requirements too, and the prison researchers treat him as a semi-colleague. After every test session, they thank Jeff for his help, and Jeff always replies, "Only a million years to go" (p. 47).

Saunders is wickedly funny about the drug testing enterprise. Jeff and the other prisoner-subjects wear a "MobiPak™" that allows researchers to administer drugs by remote control. Most of the drugs are designed to increase well-being. They are aimed at reducing social anxiety ("ChatEase™"), elevating diction and vocabulary ("Verbaluce™"), and intensifying experiences ("Vivistef™").

An exception is "Darkenfloxx™." Even brief exposure to a low dose makes you feel "the worst you have ever felt, times ten" (p. 56). Darkenfloxx is used in a test of ED289/ 90, an experimental drug that affects the amount of love people feel for each other. The researchers brag to Jeff about the experimental drug's potential: "What a fantastic game changer. Say someone can't love? Now he or she can. Say someone loves too much? Or loves someone deemed unsuitable by his or her caregiver? We can tone that shit right down" (p. 37).

Exposed to ED289/90, Jeff, two other male prisoners, and two female prisoners exhibit the desired behavior, falling in and out of love as the dosage is manipulated. The researchers are thrilled, but to measure the drug's full impact they perform another test. The test evaluates whether subjects receiving ED289/90 retain any affection for their lovers after the drug is withdrawn. As part of the experiment, Jeff is asked to give one of the two women prisoners Darkenfloxx. Jeff refuses, saying his choice would be purely random because he now feels neutral toward both women.

After observing the same behavior in the other trial subjects, the investigators are satisfied that ED289/90 has no residual effects. But the next day they tell Jeff that the "Three Horsemen of Anality" overseeing the research have insisted on another verification procedure (p. 66). With Jeff watching, researchers will administer Darkenfloxx to one of the women, Heather. To confirm that Jeff feels nothing special for the woman he formerly loved, researchers will observe what Jeff says when this occurs.

This time, however, Jeff refuses to go along. Although he doesn't feel particularly attracted to Heather he knows he doesn't want to be part of giving Darkenfloxx to anyone. But the researchers put pressure on Jeff to acquiesce. They describe Heather's villainous past, then threaten to take away Jeff's Skype visits with his mother. Jeff reluctantly agrees to participate.

When the test is performed, Jeff has the expected reaction. Although he is disturbed by what Heather is going through, he doesn't say anything suggesting that he has special feelings for her. Instead, his sorrow seems to reflect "pretty much basic human feeling" (p. 70).

Then Heather breaks off a chair leg and uses it to kill herself. The researchers are upset by this, but not upset enough to call off the test. They bring in the second woman, Rachel, and prepare to give her Darkenfloxx. This time, however, the researchers cannot persuade Jeff to utter the requisite "acknowledge."

To get around Jeff's opposition, the researchers fax their superiors for a consent waiver. While they are busy with this, Jeff decides to escape. "If I wasn't here to describe it, they wouldn't do it" (p. 77), he reasons. But the facility is secure; there is no way out. Then Jeff finds the remote that controls drug administration to the subjects. He releases the Darkenfloxx in his own MobiPak and, as he puts it, "sail[s] right out through the roof" (p. 79). When a kind voice asks if he wants to come back, he declines: "no thanks, I've had enough" (p. 80).

Jeff has to die to escape from Spiderhead. In choosing self-sacrifice, he proves himself morally superior to his scientist-captors. Jeff won't let the researchers force him to endanger another person, no matter how horrible her past sins. Jeff takes control of the situation, using a research drug to advance his own objectives rather than those of the researchers. In the end, the prisoner with a violent past is the person we admire.

UNTRUSTWORTHY SUBJECTS

Although fictional subjects are usually the heroes in these stories, not every fictional subject is virtuous. Subjects have their own agendas, which often differ from those of the researchers. Fiction can reveal a darker or selfish side to research participants.

In chapter 4, I describe real-life examples of subjects who surreptitiously violated research rules. David Gilbert's story about Billy Schine includes a colorful example of such a subject. Described as having a "Ph.D. in guinea pig," Rodney Letts considers himself an expert with valuable advice for the new study recruits. During their ride to the drug testing unit, he gives Billy and the other volunteers a warning:

> However you're feeling, really lousy, say, just keep your mouth shut. Don't tell them anything, especially if you're feeling fucked. That's a rookie mistake. Because then they get all nervous and they'll send you home early and pay you less than full. Best to keep the major side effects quiet and let the blood do the talking. They just care about your blood anyway. Oh, they'll pretend to be interested in your head but [tapping his inner arm] all they want is right here. (pp. 47–48)

Although Rodney knows more about the testing process than the new recruits do, he is also quite pathetic. He looks terrible, because he is experiencing the aftereffects of being in too many studies. He has also been drinking vinegar and using all sorts of other unappealing remedies to cleanse his system. Taking pity on Rodney, Billy slips his own urine specimen to Rodney so that he can pass the study screening tests.

Rodney is just one of several volunteers in *The Normals* who don't behave like model subjects. These volunteers misbehave in myriad ways. They fake symptoms and try to scare the new recruits by telling exaggerated war stories about previous trial experiences. They prey on a fellow subject who is obviously mentally disturbed.

The only woman in the group, Gretchen, is also the only person who mentions altruism as a motivation for enrolling in the study. But even Gretchen later admits: "you don't do something like this without knowing you're getting a good story. The story is the biggest perk" (p. 310). When she discovers that drug testing is actually too boring to furnish a good story, she decides to spice things up by sleeping with seven of the male volunteers.

UNTRUSTWORTHY RESEARCHERS

Although subjects in *The Normals* don't always behave as they should, the researchers are even worse. Billy almost dies at the hand of researchers pursuing their pet project. This is a common dynamic in research stories. Fictional subjects may have their faults, but fictional scientists have even more of them. Researchers in *Frankenstein, Flowers for Algernon, The Normals,* "Escape from Spiderhead," *Wit,* and *Miss Evers' Boys* are all less honorable than the subjects they study. At best, researchers in these stories are flawed individuals with all-too-human problems. Sometimes they are worse than that: they cut corners, pursue their own agendas, and behave in clearly unethical ways.

Like their subjects, fictional researchers are often troubled souls with personal and professional problems. In some stories, a researcher learns from the encounter with subjects, becoming a better person by the end of the story. Researchers and subjects form relationships, and researchers begin to see the world through subjects' eyes. Some researchers gain wisdom through becoming subjects themselves.

In her 2011 novel *State of Wonder*,[12] Ann Patchett writes about an unlikable researcher who becomes more appealing over time. Dr. Annick Swenson is a no-nonsense investigator who intimidates just about everyone, including her research subjects. In this case, the subjects are members of the Lakashi, an isolated tribe in the Amazon.

Swenson is not only a bully; she is deceptive. For many years, she has been concealing the true nature of her research from her drug company funders. People at the drug company think she is studying whether the ingredients in a particular tree bark can extend women's fertility until late in life. (The Lakashi women don't seem to go through menopause.) Though it's true that she is examining that question, Swenson's greater interest is in investigating the bark's antimalarial effects. She hopes to develop a malaria vaccine that could help thousands of people in low-income countries.

Swenson may have a worthy research goal, but her research methods are questionable. To induce the Lakashi women to accept vaginal swabs and other study procedures, Swenson engages in "tireless cajoling and gift giving" (p. 214). Rather than seeking the Lakashi men's informed consent to malaria exposure, researchers working under Swenson's supervision obtain their cooperation by giving them Cokes.

Swenson is unapologetic about her treatment of subjects. "I tamed them," she tells a visitor, apparently "taking not the least discomfort in the word" (pp. 214–15). Another researcher on the team has a darker view of her tactics: "I cannot imagine how terrified they must have been of her to have gone along with it" (p. 262). And although the Lakashi tolerate Swenson's actions, they don't invite her to share food or join in their ceremonies.

Yet Swenson and her team aren't all bad. Committed scientists, they are willing to bear the same research burdens they impose on the Lakashi. The researchers expose themselves to malaria to evaluate the effects of the bark, and seventy-three-year-old Swenson goes even further: to test the bark's fertility effects, she herself tries to become pregnant. She succeeds, but the pregnancy is physically difficult and Swenson suffers severe weakness and fatigue. Then the fetus dies, and Swenson needs a C-section to remove it. When asked why she didn't use someone else as a research subject, Swenson invokes ethics: "I developed this drug. If I believe in it, and I clearly do, I should be willing to test it on myself" (p. 247).

Self-experimentation teaches Swenson something important about the potential effects of a fertility-extending drug. Swenson says, "I am glad to have conducted this research on myself because it makes me realize something I might not have otherwise taken into account: women past a certain age are simply not meant to carry children" (p. 248). Before the pregnancy, Swenson never felt her age. Now she feels older than her years. Swenson sees the adverse effects as rightful punishment for "straying into the biological territory of the young" (p. 249).

In *State of Wonder*, an obsessed and manipulative scientist is transformed into someone less disturbing. Swenson deserves criticism for taking advantage of her vulnerable subjects and for mistreating many other characters in the novel. Yet Swenson's own sacrifices make her a more attractive figure. She is working toward a laudable research goal. And she subscribes to a version of equal treatment, exposing herself and her scientific colleagues to many of the same risks and indignities the Lakashi experience.

Swenson is at least partly redeemed by becoming a research subject.

Researcher Ian Ogelvie doesn't self-experiment, but bonding with a subject helps him become a more honorable person. Ian, a character in Robert Cohen's 2001 novel *Inspired Sleep*,[13] is a rather arrogant young scientist who is struggling with both personal and professional setbacks. An apartment fire destroyed his possessions and he is sleeping on his sister's sofa bed. He is also trying to recover from a breakup with a woman he loved. Ian is attracted to another young scientist in the lab, but she isn't interested, in part because she is sleeping with the department chair.

Ian was once considered a "comer, a hot young thing" (p. 40) in experimental psychology. But his experiments have stopped working and he is having trouble putting together his next grant proposal. Hoping for "a fast result" (p. 396) that he can publish, he conducts a secret sleep experiment. The subject is Bonnie Saks, an insomniac whose personal life is in shambles too.

Ian tells Bonnie she is receiving an investigational drug for her insomnia. But she is really taking sugar pills, for Ian is in fact studying the placebo effect. As the study progresses, Ian and Bonnie develop a sort of friendship. Ian is becoming disillusioned with the career he has chosen, and he feels bad about lying to Bonnie. He discovers that his department head and other colleagues are engaged in all sorts of misconduct, including shady drug studies involving prisoners. In disgust, Ian resigns from his position. By the novel's end, Bonnie has straightened out her life, and, as he heads to India to study alternative medicine, Ian is hoping to do the same.

An imperfect researcher also shows up in Christopher Robinson and Gavin Kovite's 2015 novel *War of the Encyclopaedists*.[14] In the novel, a troubled graduate school dropout named Hal Corderoy enrolls in a two-week sleep study to earn some much-needed cash. Another graduate student, Garret from MIT, is conducting the study.

Hal thinks Garret is an arrogant snob. In his "Subjective Study Record," Hal describes Garret as "kind of a dick" (p. 396). The study itself does nothing to improve Hal's attitude. He is confined in a windowless hospital room where researchers manipulate light levels to alter his sleep-wake cycles. He is also deprived of cigarettes and alcohol, which makes him miserable. He is particularly annoyed when Garret shows up smelling of nicotine.

Being in the study is quite tedious as well. Permitted to bring only one book, Hal chose *Endurance*, the story of Ernest Shackleton's ill-fated Antarctic expedition. It seems to Hal that he is enduring the same things the explorers did—unappetizing food, disorientation, and detachment from ordinary life. Desperate for distraction, Hal closely observes Garret and the other staff members who come into his room. They may be watching him, he thinks, but "the watched can watch as well" (p. 403).

As time passes, Hal gradually changes his opinion of Garret. One day he sees Garret trying but failing to flirt with the study nurse. Then, while Hal is taking tests that measure his reaction times, something goes wrong with the computer. The space bar malfunctions, and Hal breaks down too. The research has taken a toll on him and he wants to quit. He begs Garret to release him from the study.

In response, Garret exposes his own anxieties. Two other subjects have already dropped out, he admits. He pleads with Hal to continue: "Please just stick it out, Hal. I need this" (p. 403). After witnessing Garret's breakdown, Hal sees that his initial impression was wrong: Garret is "not an asshole, he's just socially awkward." Garret's good looks and nice clothes misled Hal. In fact, Hal thinks, Garret is "even more socially inept than I am" (p. 404).

Garret proves to be an insecure and fretful human being, not the confident elitist Hal took him to be. Seeing Garret as an ordinary guy with ordinary problems helps Hal settle down. He resolves to make it through the study, and he does. In this story, the researcher who reveals his vulnerabilities to his subject becomes a person worthy of understanding and compassion.

The most popular targets in fictional critiques are drug company researchers. But writers also find fault with researchers in other settings. In *Wit*, for example, Edson raises questions about the morality of academic researchers. The suspect researchers in *Inspired Sleep* are highly regarded academics (although the hospital they work in has just been bought by a corporation). *Miss Evers' Boys* takes on the government-sponsored researchers who carried out the Tuskegee syphilis study. And an experienced volunteer in *The Normals* warns other subjects, "the government can fuck you up" (p. 186).

Whether part of the drug industry or not, researchers rarely come off well in these stories. Writers remove scientists from their usual pedestal, putting them on a level at or below the subjects they study. But when researchers show their human side, they become people we can care about. Researchers are transformed through interactions and relationships with subjects, or by becoming subjects themselves. In fiction, it is usually subjects who rescue researchers, rather than the reverse.

RESEARCH ETHICS AND OVERSIGHT

Ethics and oversight are in the background of many research stories. Writers tend to portray ethical and regulatory standards as well intended but ineffective. Fictional researchers disregard what they consider to be unreasonable demands from FDA officials, ethics review committees, and lawyers. Rogue scientists like Annick Swenson in *State of Wonder* and Ian Ogelvie in *Inspired Sleep* conceal their work from authorities, claiming that secrecy is necessary to allow their important projects to go forward. A member of Swenson's team explains their questionable conduct this way: "It's good to get out of the American medical system from time to time. . . . It frees a person up, makes them think about what's possible" (p. 295).

At the same time, the writers' allegiance is to subjects put at risk by outlaw scientists. Writers see weaknesses in oversight, but they also see a need for it. Researchers who disregard the rules are often punished—in *White Noise*, Mr. Gray gets shot; in *State of Wonder*, Dr. Swenson loses her health; and in *The Normals*, researchers conducting an unauthorized study get fired.

Informed consent is the ethics topic that appears most often in research stories. Writers usually portray consent discussions as mere formalities, mandatory rituals that neither researchers nor subjects take seriously. This doesn't necessarily mean that the writers think informed consent is unimportant. But many do seem to think that current practice fails to promote choice in the ways that it should.

In *The Normals*, Billy Schine is involved in two meaningless consent discussions. Early in the novel, Billy becomes impatient when a doctor describes the drug trial Billy plans to join. Eager to sign the form, he urges the doctor to skip the study information. Later, when Billy volunteers for a different (unauthorized) experiment, he is even less interested in study facts. When the researcher starts explaining what will happen, Billy interrupts and says: "I don't want to know anything. I don't want any information. I'm sick of being informed. I'm just going to stay ignorant and do what you guys tell me to do" (p. 347).

Similarly, Bonnie Saks, the research subject in *Inspired Sleep*, pays little attention to what Ian, the investigator, tells her about his study. Her mind is elsewhere. She is thinking about what the sleep lab looks like, what is on Ian's mind, and how she is dressed—she wears socks in bed to hide her unattractive feet. After a bit, Bonnie tells Ian not to bother with the study explanation. "I'm just as happy being ignorant of the details," she says (p. 204). What does bother her is Ian's formality and failure to call her by name.

In *Wit*, the research subject is distracted during the consent discussion too, but by something more serious. As I discussed in chapter 3, many seriously ill patients don't understand central facts about the trials they join. Playwright Edson shows how this can happen. Vivian Bearing is not really listening as researcher Dr. Kelekian describes the cancer study he wants her to join. Instead, she is contemplating his word choices ("insidious" adenocarcinoma and "pernicious" side effects) as well as the reading about cancer that she ought to do.

Vivian signs the consent form without really understanding what she has agreed to. After Kelekian leaves, she acknowledges her poor performance: "I should have asked more questions, because I know there's going to be a test. I have cancer, insidious cancer, with pernicious side effects—no, the *treatment* has pernicious side effects" (p. 12). Even a highly educated, extremely intelligent person is unable to concentrate on study information after receiving a diagnosis of advanced cancer.

Some stories feature consent discussions in the context of research involving characters with mental disabilities. Matthew Thomas's 2014 novel *We Are Not Ourselves*[15] portrays dementia research from the perspective of a subject and his wife. In the novel, a family saga, the husband is Ed Leary, a neuroscientist specializing in psychopharmacology. Early in his career, he turns down a high-paying industry job, as well as a prestigious academic position, because he prefers to teach working-class students at a community college.

In a twist of fate, Leary himself becomes a subject in a psychopharmacology study. He is diagnosed with Alzheimer's disease, and his wife, Eileen, arranges for him to join a study evaluating a potential Alzheimer's drug. Eileen, a nurse, sees the study as the only possible way to slow down his mental deterioration. She wants him in the study even though he "would be helping the industry he had balked at working for, and he wouldn't get a dime for it" (p. 324).

Eileen is acutely aware of Ed's deficits, but she also knows that he still understands a lot. She's irritated when the investigators ask her to sign a form saying that Ed is incapable of making his own research decisions, "because Ed so clearly understood what they were telling him, probably understood it better than they did themselves" (p. 325). And he does understand. During a follow-up visit, he tells Eileen he feels like one of the rats he used to study. But he isn't upset by it. "I can be the rat after all these years," he says. "Maybe it will help someone." When Eileen insists that the drug might also help him, he answers: "I'm not the point of this. This is a trial. Other people are the point of this" (p. 332).

Ed demonstrates his understanding to the researchers too. When a study doctor asks Ed if he wants Eileen to have the power to make decisions for him, Ed laughs and asks the doctor if he is married. When the doctor nods, Ed says, "Then it won't surprise you to hear that my wife has been calling the shots as long as we've been married" (p. 325). The doctor chuckles and checks the box to confirm that Ed has the capacity to designate a surrogate decision-maker.

Although Ed is cheerful during this discussion, Eileen is struggling to keep her composure. She marvels at Ed's ability to be so charming in what seems to her a heart-breaking situation. As she watches Ed sign the form, she can barely keep from crying: "he started his signature an inch above where he should have and angled it down and through the line in a way that made it look as if he was falling down as he did it" (p. 325).

Years later, after Ed's death, Eileen has second thoughts about the research. It was a three-year study, but she "kept him on the medicine another two, until it was too hard to get him to swallow the pills. It wasn't entirely to spite her that he resisted: he had an instinctual fear of choking" (pp. 568–69). Ed's body had also became quite rigid over time, which made him difficult to manage and contributed to his placement in a nursing facility. Rigidity was one of the drug's known side effects, and Eileen wonders whether the drug was the cause in Ed's case. It wasn't clear that Ed had benefited from the drug, and it might have shortened the time he could be cared for at home.

Although Eileen has some regrets about the study, she made the choice to enroll Ed as a loving surrogate, and Ed himself seemed to know what he was getting into. By contrast, *Flowers for Algernon* describes a clearly deficient consent process. When the lead researcher warns Charlie that the experiment could fail or leave him worse off, Charlie is unconcerned. As he writes in his journal, "I ain't afraid of nothing. Im very strong and I always do good and beside I got my luky rabits foot and I never breakd a mirrir in my life" (p. 11). The researchers realize that Charlie cannot consent for himself, so they look for a surrogate decision maker. Although Charlie's family abandoned him when he was a teenager, the researchers are able to track down his sister. She hasn't seen him for years, yet she consents to his participation.

Flowers for Algernon, Wit, and *We Are Not Ourselves* depict the consent process from the perspectives of vulnerable subjects and their families. In *Flowers for Algernon*, neither Charlie nor his sister makes an informed choice about the experiment. In *Wit*, Vivian Bearing signs a consent form without knowing very much about the cancer study she is joining. And in *We Are Not Ourselves*, Eileen appears unduly optimistic that the study will help her husband. Ironically, the study participant with the most accurate understanding in these stories is the Alzheimer's patient who was once a researcher himself.

QUESTIONABLE RESEARCH GOALS

Fictional works often raise questions about the value of certain research objectives. Scientists in some research stories, such as *White Noise* and "Escape from Spiderhead," are working on measures to enhance life rather than to treat disease. Their research seeks to alter what have always been inescapable human challenges, like facing mortality and finding the right person to love. Many writers of such stories are skeptical of research endeavors of this kind—they don't seem to approve of them. Putting their views into story form is a compelling way to convey what is disturbing about the research.

No one does this better than George Saunders in "Escape from Spiderhead." Research at the prison is all about enhancement. For example, when researchers administer one of the test drugs, subjects looking at an ordinary garden feel great wonder, sensing "the eternal in the ephemeral." A researcher explains that such a drug would be useful to people saddled with tedious chores: "say a guy has to stay up late guarding a perimeter. Or is at school waiting for his kid and gets bored. But there's some nature nearby?" (p. 46)

As I described earlier, the main drug being tested in Saunders's story, ED289/90, is designed to control the love one person feels for another. The researchers are very excited about this drug: Besides offering help in the romance department, ED289/90 could improve international relations. Giving it to soldiers could put an end to war, a researcher declares, or "sure as heck slow it down! Suddenly the soldiers on both sides start fucking. Or, at a lower dosage, feeling super-fond" (p. 58).

The researchers in "Escape from Spiderhead" see these as valuable goals that justify what they do to Jeff and the other subjects. "Do the math," says a researcher—"a few minutes of unpleasantness" in exchange for "years of relief for literally thousands of underloving or overloving folks" (p. 75). To the scientists, the agony produced by Darkenfloxx and even the death of a subject are well worth the cost. But the story's conclusion exposes the research as unjustified and corrupt.

Gary Shteyngart offers another skeptical take on enhancement research in his 2011 novel *Super Sad True Love Story*.[16] This time the research goal is immortality, and the setting is the near future. Thirty-nine-year old Lenny Abramov opens the novel with a declaration: "I am never going to die" (p. 3). Lenny is the "Life Lovers Outreach Coordinator" of "Post-Human Services," part of a huge corporate conglomerate. Lenny's company is developing indefinite life-extension technology[17] for attractive "High Net Worth" ("HNW") individuals (p. 5). The company sees itself as responding to an urgent human problem. As Lenny explains, "each peaceful, natural death at age eighty-one is a tragedy without compare" (p. 4).

The company's life-extending technology is still in the research phase, but many HNW individuals are eager to be part of the testing. Just 18 percent of applicants are accepted, however. Besides the physical assessments, applicants have to pass a series of cognitive tests, like the "willingness-to-persevere-in-difficult-conditions test" (p. 125). As Lenny observes, "You had to prove that you were worthy of cheating death at Post-Human Services" (p. 153).

The CEO, Joshie Goldmann, is the biggest user of his company's products. Although Joshie is in his seventies, his body has been "reverse-engineered into a thick young mass of tendons and forward motion" (p. 217). His youthful appearance helps him seduce the young woman Lenny loves.

But Joshie's good fortune doesn't last. At the end of *Super Sad True Love Story*, we learn that "dechronification" has failed. The technology produced complications that couldn't be reversed. A twitching and drooling Joshie explains: "Our genocidal war on free radicals proved more damaging than helpful, hurting cellular metabolism, robbing the body of control. In the end, nature simply would not yield" (p. 329).

"Escape from Spiderhead" and *Super Sad True Love Story* are dystopian fantasies about where enhancement technologies could lead us. By contrast, it is easy to envision a present-day enhancement study like the one that takes place in Kate Fodor's 2011 play *Rx*.[18]

The study subject in *Rx* is Meena, a poet who supports herself by working as managing editor of *American Cattle & Swine Magazine*. Meena is miserable at her job. At a study screening interview, she admits to crying about her situation at least twice a day. Meena wants desperately to enroll in a trial of an investigational drug for "workplace depression." As Phil, a study doctor, explains, the company is developing the drug "for patients with a household income of at least $65,000" (lower-income workers don't have insurance).

Meena is thrilled to be admitted to the trial. For a time, however, the drug doesn't seem to work. Still, the trial has a positive impact. As Meena and Phil get to know each other, they develop a personal relationship. They become lovers and make plans to leave their jobs for something more fulfilling.

But then Meena starts liking her job at the magazine. She becomes obsessed with her work projects and has little time for Phil. The relationship deteriorates, and then Phil loses his job because his superiors find out about the romance— Phil wrote poems and drew little hearts on Meena's research chart. Rather than conducting the independent data review the FDA requires when violations like this occur, company officials shut down the trial. The company has invested $49 million in drug development, but now nothing will come of it. And although Meena was convinced the drug was working, she was actually in the placebo group.

Saunders, Shteyngart, and Fodor use the research enterprise as a setting for cultural critique. They don't buy the drug company PR and media hype about the miracles research has in store for us. They don't like the idea that science can rescue us from every human problem. They fear that enhancement measures will make human life shallow and uninteresting. They also doubt that such measures will be safe and effective. In *Super Sad True Love Story*, interventions that at first seem to work later prove to have dangerous effects. In *Rx*, a subject who thinks the investigational drug is working is actually taking a placebo. In these research stories, as well as in *White Noise* and *State of Wonder*, the scientific pursuit of enhancement is both risky and misguided.

THE MESSAGES OF RESEARCH FICTION

Researchers and ethicists ought to read the work of the talented and discerning writers discussed in this chapter. Their research stories are captivating and beautifully written. Fiction brings research, as well as research ethics, to life. Otherwise unnoticed events and issues become visible when creative writers address human subject research. Unsettling aspects of research are hauntingly exposed when seen through the eyes of fictional subjects.

Works of fiction present a rich picture of the research enterprise, one in which subjects play a much greater role than is generally understood. In fiction, subjects are interesting and multifaceted, and so are researchers. In fiction, research involves complicated relationships, deep emotions, good and bad motivations, and unexpected outcomes. In fiction, research interactions exhibit the same characteristics that other human interactions do.

Research is also messy in novels, short stories, and plays. Reading this work, we find all kinds of "unscientific" behavior. Friendship, romance, generosity, and soul-searching appear in research fiction, as do cynicism, opportunism, deception, bullying, and hidden agendas.

Fiction is an antidote to the myopic and impoverished conception of human research that prevails in the professional literature. Research stories offer insights into why people volunteer for studies and why measures like informed consent are so often ineffective. Stories illuminate subjects' thinking as well as the power dynamics that affect their research experiences. And in stories, research observations go two ways. While researchers are evaluating their subjects, subjects are evaluating their researchers.

Fiction communicates the views of a perceptive and influential segment of the public. And the authors I discuss present an unflattering picture of research. In their work, self-serving scientists violate scientific and ethical norms to achieve their goals. Preoccupied with their own concerns, researchers take advantage of subjects. Subjects must be on guard for such behavior, for rules and procedures designed to protect them often fall short.

The work of these creative writers challenges the feel-good research narratives that populate the professional and mass media. Although the stories aren't real, they bring to light real unease about the research endeavor. Fictional research stories can help scientists and ethicists understand that unease.

NOTES

1. Many films also explore human subject research. For examples, see Henri Colt, Silvia Quadrelli, and Friedman Lester, eds., *The Picture of Health: Medical Ethics and the Movies* (New York: Oxford University Press, 2011); Sandra Shapshay, ed., *Bioethics at the Movies* (Baltimore: Johns Hopkins University Press, 2009).
2. Mary Shelley, *Frankenstein* (New York: Signet Classics, 1963).
3. Harold Bloom, "Afterword," in ibid., 199–210, 202.
4. Don DeLillo, *White Noise* (New York: Penguin Books, 1986).
5. David Gilbert, *The Normals* (New York: Bloomsbury, 2004).
6. Daniel Keyes, *Flowers for Algernon* (New York: Harcourt, 2004). The novel is based on a short story that Keyes published in 1959. It has been adapted for the theater, television, and film, most notably in the award-winning 1968 movie *Charly*.
7. Charlie identifies with Algernon throughout the book. At various points, he complains about Algernon's mistreatment. For example, in their tests of Algernon's abilities, researchers use food to motivate the mouse. Charlie writes in his journal, "I don't think its right to make you pass a test to eat." Ibid., 31. In *The Normals*, Billy Schine also feels a bond with the animal subjects housed in the same research center the human subjects occupy.
8. Margaret Edson, *Wit* (New York: Faber & Faber, 1999). The play also goes by the name *W;t*. Vivian Bearing is an authority on John Donne's Holy Sonnets, and in the play she recalls a lesson about the importance of using a comma rather than a semicolon in the final line of Donne's poem "Death Be Not Proud."
9. David Feldshuh, *Miss Evers' Boys* (New York: Dramatists Play Service, 1995). For description of the actual study, see James H. Jones, *Bad Blood: The Tuskegee Syphilis Experiment*, expanded ed. (New York: Free Press, 1993).
10. For a review of the evidence on Rivers's role in the study, see Susan Reverby, *Examining Tuskegee: The Infamous Syphilis Study and Its Legacy* (Chapel Hill: University of North Carolina Press, 2009).

11. George Saunders, "Escape from Spiderhead," in *Tenth of December* (New York: Random House, 2013).

12. Ann Patchett, *State of Wonder* (New York: HarperCollins, 2011).

13. Robert Cohen, *Inspired Sleep* (New York: Scribner, 2001).

14. Christopher Robinson and Gavin Kovite, *War of the Encyclopaedists* (New York: Scribner, 2015).

15. Matthew Thomas, *We Are Not Ourselves* (New York: Simon & Schuster, 2014).

16. Gary Shteyngart, *Super Sad True Love Story* (New York: Random House, 2011).

17. In the novel's acknowledgments, Shteyngart says he was influenced by the ideas of Ray Kurzweil and Aubrey de Grey, who argue that science can and should seek to prevent human aging and death. See Ray Kurzweil, *The Singularity is Near: When Humans Transcend Biology* (New York: Penguin Group, 2005); Aubrey de Grey, *Ending Aging: The Rejuvenation Breakthroughs That Could Reverse Human Aging in Our Lifetime* (New York: St. Martin's, 2007).

18. Kate Fodor, *Rx* (New York: WME Entertainment, 2011). Recent fiction also raises compelling questions about whether human cloning is a defensible research goal. Two of the best examples are Caryl Churchill's play *A Number* (London: Nick Hern Books, 2002) and Kazuo Ishiguro's novel *Never Let Me Go* (New York: Alfred A. Knopf, 2005).

How to Hear Subjects

∎◻∎

RESEARCH EXPERTS OFTEN SPEAK OF research subjects as partners in an enterprise that will someday allow people to live longer and better lives. But talk of this partnership is more promotional than descriptive. Subjects have relatively little power in the research world. Ethicist Alexander Capron hit the mark in calling it "wishful thinking to suppose that most of the people on whom research is conducted today in the United States are on a par with—that is, are co-equal participants with—the research team and sponsors."[1]

During the 1970s, researchers and government officials began to accept certain research "outsiders"—nonscientists and members of the general public—as colleagues in ethics and policy activities. Research oversight rules and professional policies now promote the involvement of those research outsiders.

The next step is to recognize the distinct contributions that experienced research subjects can make to ethics and oversight. In many respects, experienced subjects are more qualified to perform the desired functions of research outsiders than are nonscientists and members of the public who have never participated in research. Experienced subjects are "sociologically and ethically 'key' informants" in the effort to provide meaningful human subject protection.[2]

THE VALUE OF SUBJECT INCLUSION: A REVIEW

Experienced subjects have a specific expertise that allows them to enrich and supplement deliberations about research ethics and policy. Research deliberations that fail to include experienced subjects are deficient, just as research deliberations that omitted scientists, physicians, or ethicists would be deficient.

Previous chapters describe in detail what experienced subjects can contribute. Experienced subjects know things about research participation that no one else knows. These include facts about what participation is really like as well as potential ethical problems with particular aspects of research. At times it is simply the case that, as one subject put it, "you can't understand it until you experience it."[3] Experienced subjects' views of ethical matters can differ from those of professionals and members of the public who have never participated in studies. The usual practice of "making up" subjects—speculating about how people experience study participation—is an unacceptable substitute for hearing from subjects themselves.[4]

Research subjects don't necessarily see research the way others think they do. For example, historians have made assumptions about subjects' experiences that have contributed to oversimplified characterizations of past research practices. Considering subjects' personal accounts can lead to more complex, and more realistic, narratives. When two contemporary scholars examined subjects' experiences in two LSD studies conducted by National Institutes of Health (NIH) researchers in the 1950s, they found that subjects "attributed a wider range of meaning to actions and events unfolding in experimental settings" than previous scholars had recognized.[5] Although testimony from one subject supported the conventional view that LSD study subjects were vulnerable and exploited, other subjects—namely, church members who volunteered as a form of religious service—believed they had been treated appropriately. This look at subjects' perceptions showed that "both types of relationships—exploitative and cooperative" existed in the decades before modern research rules came into being.[6]

As this example suggests, more information about subject perspectives won't necessarily support more restrictive research rules or practices. It's true that such information can point to a need for stronger protective measures to address previously unrecognized burdens on subjects—but information on subject perspectives can also suggest that certain protective measures are unnecessary. Finding out what participants think can help researchers and institutional review boards (IRBs) "avoid rejecting study procedures as harmful, when in fact prospective participants see them as posing little if any [risk], and evaluate the benefits as clearly outweighing the risks."[7]

People who study subject perspectives see their work as essential to a morally defensible human research system. When traditional experts control rules and ethical decisions, "the scholarly community and IRB members risk treating subjects as 'research material' rather than as moral agents with the right to judge the ethicality of investigative procedures in which they are asked to participate."[8] According to a report on HIV prevention studies by the Joint United Nations Programme on HIV/AIDS (UNAIDS), meaningful engagement with research stakeholders like experienced subjects promotes respect, trust, agreement, and understanding in the research endeavor. The report declares that prevention studies "cannot succeed" without the engagement of these stakeholders.[9]

Statements like these are common in the published literature. Scholarly and organizational support for subject inclusion isn't difficult to find. But real change requires more than words—it requires action. Effective implementation is the key to meaningful subject inclusion.

PUTTING INCLUSION INTO PRACTICE

Subject inclusion has two components: procedural and substantive. The procedural component requires decision makers to appoint experienced subjects to groups that oversee research as well as groups that develop individual studies and research policy advice. The substantive component requires decision makers to take subject perspectives into account when developing and evaluating research policies and practices. Below I describe how to address both inclusion components.

Inclusion in Research Oversight

To promote "complete and adequate review of research ethics activities," federal regulations require each IRB to include not only researchers and clinicians but also nonscientists and people unaffiliated with the research institution.[10] The regulations fail to assign to particular IRB members a responsibility to represent subjects, but many nonscientist and unaffiliated members see subject representation as one of their primary responsibilities.[11] For example, most of the unaffiliated members interviewed for one study said that "their responsibility was to take the perspective of potential research participants when reading protocols and consent forms."[12] Another team that interviewed unaffiliated members found that most saw their role as "representing or giving a voice to human subjects."[13]

The ethical and regulatory presumption is that all IRB members will consider how subjects could experience study participation, and empirical evidence suggests that members do try to put themselves in the subjects' position.[14] But for the most part, their judgments rest on speculation. For example, most of the forty IRB members interviewed for one project said that they "had little knowledge of the values, expectations, and needs of those whom they are charged to protect."[15] Few of the nonscientist and unaffiliated IRB members interviewed for another project said they had experience as either a research subject or a patient with serious illness.[16]

When sociologist Laura Stark observed multiple meetings of three IRBs, she found that all members, scientists and nonscientists alike, relied on "their own life experiences" to decide how study procedures would affect potential study participants. Members developed their views on subject perspectives by envisioning how people like their students, parents, friends, and neighbors would respond to various research issues. Instead of looking to experienced subjects for guidance, IRB members "imagined the people who featured in their own lives as stand-ins for research participants."[17]

A few advisory groups have recognized the drawbacks of relying on conjecture. In 2001, an Institute of Medicine committee evaluating the US subject protection system urged institutions to include more experienced research subjects in review and oversight activities. The committee recommended that IRBs involve experienced subjects or other individuals "who genuinely understand and represent the perspectives of particular subject populations."[18] The organization that accredits human subject protection programs includes in its standard on IRB membership the expectation that an IRB will have "one or more members who represent the general perspective of participants."[19] According to that organization's president, "current or former research subjects" have the necessary understanding to represent those perspectives.[20]

At least one research center has arranged for actual subject representation on its IRB. At Fort Detrick, a US Army facility in Maryland, soldiers training to be medics can choose to become medical research volunteer subjects. From time to time, these individuals are invited to participate in studies conducted at the facility's Infectious Disease Institute. Volunteers are not obligated to participate in research, although they must attend informational sessions about studies in need of subjects. One volunteer also serves on the research unit's IRB. Ethicist Jonathan Moreno writes that subject representation on the IRB is one reason that volunteers at Fort Detrick are "arguably the least exploited human experimental subjects in the country, if not the world."[21]

Besides appointing experienced subjects to IRBs, institutions could promote more informed and defensible subject protection programs by involving subjects in other ethics oversight activities. For example, committees that monitor the safety of ongoing human studies could include experienced subjects.[22] Research oversight programs could establish advisory groups made up of subjects with different types of research experience. Programs could then call on advisory group members with relevant experience when specific study issues come up.[23] Educational sessions for IRB members, IRB staff, and researchers could include presentations by experienced subjects on what it was like to be in different types of studies (see chapter 2).

Research protection programs could also seek feedback from subjects in studies at their institutions. Programs could survey former and current subjects about their experiences.[24] Feedback from experienced subjects would help IRBs learn about problems that need attention. It would also enable institutions to design educational sessions that address subjects' genuine concerns.[25]

Inclusion in the Research Process

Institutional review boards and other oversight groups evaluate completed research proposals. Making the revisions these groups call for can be time-consuming and disruptive for researchers. If experienced subjects are enlisted to help with proposal development, however, subjects' perspectives can more easily be taken into account, reducing the need for such revisions. Also, through this approach, people with the greatest impact on subjects—the research team—are directly exposed to subjects' viewpoints. Helping researchers see studies from the subjects' point of view increases the chance that they will design and conduct studies with subject perspectives in mind.

During the 1980s, researchers and government officials began including patients, patient advocates, and community members in planning, implementing, and evaluating the merit of studies, as well as in setting research priorities and in research policy activities. The practice has continued, developing into the activities now known as community engagement, community consultation, participatory research, patient-centered research, and deliberative democratic proceedings on research issues.[26]

The primary motivation for including patients and community members is to improve the quality and value of health research. Researchers and policy officials are trying to make research more responsive to patients' actual needs. They also hope to increase recruitment and retention of study subjects and produce maximum health benefits from research investments.[27] Research professionals portray patients and other potential study participants as experts with knowledge relevant to research improvements.[28] They believe that researchers and policymakers can learn from these lay experts, just as they learn from traditional research experts.

Supporters of patient and community engagement say the practice can advance ethical and regulatory objectives too. For example, an NIH statement describes how engagement can promote ethical research: "Engagement creates opportunities to improve the consent process, identify ethical pitfalls, and create processes for resolving ethical problems when they arise."[29] One study team reported that community-based participation "facilitated the sensitive and respectful treatment and positive experiences" of women enrolled in a randomized clinical trial.[30] Other supporters of engagement refer to an "overarching ethical mandate for patient participation in [designing and conducting] research as a manifestation of the 'democratization' of the research process."[31]

What is missing from the literature on patient-centered research, community engagement, and similar models is explicit recognition of the singular contributions that people with actual research experience can make. Experienced subjects know how the research process works, including problems that can arise in that process. They know about practices that promote subject well-being and practices that make participation harder than it has to be.

A variety of improvements could come from consulting experienced subjects. Researchers sensitive to subject perspectives will minimize demands for study visits, tests, procedures, and time imposed on participants.[32] They will consider subjects' preferences about scheduling and other logistical matters.[33] They will measure outcomes that are important to patients, such as the discomfort associated with experimental treatments, in addition to traditional laboratory and clinical outcomes.[34] They will recruit skilled, organized, and attentive staff members who treat subjects with courtesy and respect. And they will adopt study methods that minimize the number of patient-subjects exposed to risky and ineffective interventions.[35]

Though patients and other community members who lack actual research experience can provide useful input on potential study improvements, their views and attitudes cannot substitute for those of experienced study subjects. Researchers and policy officials involved in the effort to incorporate patient and community perspectives should recognize the special status of people with real research experience and act to ensure that such experienced participants are part of that effort.

Inclusion in Ethical and Policy Deliberations

The voices of experienced subjects belong in deliberations over specific ethics and policy matters too. Bringing experienced subjects into the research mainstream would allow researchers, ethicists, and officials to discover what subjects themselves think people should know before enrolling in research, as well as subjects' views on acceptable risk and other ethical and regulatory issues.[36] Input from experienced subjects could lead to more meaningful and effective guidelines and regulations for human subject research.

For example, advisory groups trying to promote informed research choices should include experienced subjects in their deliberations. Everyone agrees that many research subjects lack a good understanding of the studies they join. Experts have made many attempts to improve this situation, without much success. A collaborative effort with experienced subjects might produce better results. People who have actually made study decisions know what was helpful and what was confusing when researchers talked with them about participation.

Experienced subjects know about measures that can help people facing research choices too. In a community survey, "talking to a study participant" was one of the respondents' top four preferred ways to learn about studies.[37] Children have recommended this as well: three-quarters of a group of children enrolled in cancer trials said they would have liked to speak to other child subjects "to help them understand what it means to be part of a study."[38] Guidelines and regulations could encourage researchers and institutions to make such opportunities available to prospective research subjects.

Experienced subjects also reveal a neglected aspect of research decision-making. Empirical data show that many patients need emotional support, as well as clear and accessible information, when choosing whether to enroll in trials. In interviews, one research group found that adult patients in trials felt that including family members and nurses in study discussions was a "highly important" source of support.[39] Another group found that parents considering enrolling their children in research studies understood randomization much better when a nurse was present during the study discussion. This finding points to "the benefits of better emotional support for parents at this difficult time, creating an environment in which parents feel empowered to speak up, ask questions, and seek clarifications."[40] Experienced study participants could help ethics advisory groups and government officials develop measures to emotionally support people confronting research choices in the midst of serious illness.

Research ethicists and policymakers should also solicit experienced subjects' views on broader issues related to research consent. We ought to know what experienced subjects think about questions like the following:

- Are current research practices defensible in light of the substantial empirical evidence that many people join studies without a good understanding of important study facts?
- If not, what should be done to address the situation?
- Should researchers be required to assess and verify prospective subjects' understanding before enrollment?[41]
- Should researchers be required to exclude prospective subjects who cannot demonstrate an adequate

understanding of the facts, even though this would make it harder to fill enrollment quotas?

Consent in comparative-effectiveness research is another policy question in need of subject input. Comparative-effectiveness research evaluates existing treatments and other medical practices to determine whether one is better than the others. Some ethicists and researchers argue that the usual informed consent requirements should not apply to this form of research because all the study interventions are already in medical use. They say that since patients in such research could receive any of the interventions as part of their ordinary medical care, the requirements for informed consent should be weakened or waived.[42] Some also argue that patients have a duty to participate in research that could improve healthcare, and thus the usual consent requirements should be relaxed.[43] Another group of ethicists and researchers, however, contends that randomization and other aspects of comparative-effectiveness research justify applying the usual consent requirements to such trials.[44]

Not enough has been done to solicit the views of experienced study subjects on these issues. Indeed, little information is available on patients' attitudes toward proposals to replace traditional consent with "largely untried practices" such as opt-out or notification procedures.[45] Data from a few general surveys and focus groups have been reported, but more information is needed. We ought to find out what experienced subjects think people should know before they are enrolled in comparative-effectiveness research. Do people who have participated in this form of research think it would be acceptable to bypass or abbreviate the usual consent requirements? What sorts of consent alternatives would be acceptable to this population? Scholars and officials cannot defensibly claim to have resolved these questions if they do not consider the views of people who know what it is like to be a subject in comparative-effectiveness research.[46]

Experienced subjects should be asked to weigh in on these and other contested research issues.[47] Deliberations on topics like payment to subjects, return of research results, and appropriate standards for surrogate decision-making should include the voices of people who have participated in research. Deliberations and decisions about study advertising and other recruitment tools, subjects' responsibilities in research, and appropriate limits on research risks should incorporate subjects' views as well.[48] Without subject input, ethical guidelines and regulatory requirements addressing these matters will lack normative legitimacy.

SUBJECT INCLUSION: THE CHALLENGES

Like any change in policy and practice, inclusion of experienced subjects will require commitment and resources. Yet subject inclusion is not a radical departure from the status quo. Many elements of subject inclusion could be put in place with relatively small adjustments to the existing system. And the move to include experienced subjects would not necessarily increase research costs. Subject recruitment and retention rates could go up in trials that take subjects' perspectives into account, thus reducing the overall costs of completing those trials.

Initiatives to include experienced subjects could have added side benefits. Long-standing efforts to involve members of the public in IRB and other research ethics activities have been less successful than many advocates for such inclusion had hoped.[49] Programs to include experienced subjects would create opportunities to promote deeper involvement of public representatives as well.

Choosing Subject Representatives

Experienced subjects participating in ethics and oversight must be capable of representing larger subject populations. Although it will sometimes be possible to include multiple subject representatives in ethics and policy deliberations, it will never be possible to capture every subject perspective. It will take thought and effort to design a process that promotes reasonable and fair representation of subjects' views.

Careful consideration must be given to the criteria for choosing subject representatives. Potential selection criteria include the range and duration of an applicant's experience as a research participant. Also important is an applicant's ability to communicate with other individuals who have been study subjects.

Compensation for subject representatives could be an important factor in attracting a diverse group of applicants. A program reliant on unpaid volunteers might attract only people who have had very positive or very negative experiences as research subjects.[50] Such a program could also have a hard time attracting a socially and economically diverse applicant group.

Finding the right subject representatives will be challenging, but the difficulties should not be exaggerated. The representation challenges resemble those that exist whenever individuals are selected for research ethics and oversight activities. Scientists, clinicians, ethicists, and members of the public deliberating about research ethics and policy issues are expected to represent large and diverse groups. The selection criteria used to promote reasonable and fair representation of other groups could be applied to promote reasonable and fair subject representation too.

Moreover, a program to include experienced subjects would create opportunities to develop more defensible selection processes for everyone participating in research ethics and oversight. Experts and members of the public sometimes are selected for IRBs and other ethics groups based on questionable criteria. For example, researchers and physicians may be chosen simply because their department heads think they need another committee assignment. Members of the public may be chosen because they happen to be neighbors or acquaintances of an existing IRB member. A move to include subjects could trigger a needed evaluation of selection criteria for all participants in research ethics and oversight groups.[51]

Procedures and Preparation

To be effective in research decision-making, experienced subjects must be full-fledged players in the process. Research professionals accustomed to control must be willing to share authority. They must respect the knowledge that experienced subjects bring to the table.

Professional dominance is a problem that often exists in research ethics groups like IRBs. Indeed, it can be a problem whenever experts and laypersons work together, as in community-engaged and patient-centered research and other efforts to involve patients and the public in health policy decisions.[52] Fortunately, there are things that can be done to reduce professional dominance.

Evidence on how to promote shared authority comes from a randomized trial evaluating public involvement in setting healthcare priorities. The trial showed that certain interventions promoted mutual influence and greater agreement among professionals and members of the public. For example, discussions moderated by a communications expert led to more deliberation and compromise than did discussions moderated by healthcare experts. Success was linked to the communication expert's efforts to encourage broad participation, solicit dissenting views, and demand clarification of technical terms. Small groups were most conducive to egalitarian discussions. Seating plans that put experts and public members next to each other, together with opportunities for informal social interaction, promoted mutual respect among group members.[53]

The research team also found that adequate training had a big role in promoting public participation in the deliberations. Members of the public gained confidence and credibility by participating in a preparation session before they met with professionals. At that session, these individuals discussed their personal experiences as patients and caregivers, which led to "a broadening of the participants' perspectives and their growing sense of a collective 'public representative' identity."[54] They also had opportunities to learn about what would happen during the later priority-setting deliberations.

People involved in community-engaged, patient-centered, and participatory research see training measures like these as prerequisites to effective inclusion.[55] Patient advocates seeking to influence research policy and practice learned this lesson early, when they first became involved in decision-making about HIV/AIDS and breast cancer research.[56] Since then, advocates representing many patient groups have developed a variety of excellent training opportunities to enhance their participation in research activities.[57]

Experienced subjects will need similar kinds of preparation and training to be effective. Yet the challenge is not as substantial as it might seem. Experienced subjects can take advantage of the educational opportunities that already exist for patient advocates and other lay participants in research activities. Personal experience as a subject is also a form of preparation for joining research activities. This experience enables subjects to enter these activities with a more extensive knowledge base than some other novices begin with. Additional training is still a good idea, but it should not be difficult to provide experienced subjects with the necessary background information for effective participation.

Measuring Subject Perspectives

Obtaining high-quality information about subject experiences will be central to many inclusion efforts. Research decisions based on subject experiences should be supported by an adequate evidentiary foundation. This means that information must be systematically gathered from a representative group of subjects.

Empirical studies are one important source of information. Surveys, questionnaires, and qualitative studies produce valuable evidence about subject perspectives. Empirical data are highly influential in other policy contexts, and they should be influential in the research policy context too.

At the same time, empirical investigations of subject perspectives present a distinct challenge. Experts designing, conducting, and interpreting the results of studies of subject perspectives are guided by their own ideas about the topic. As one social scientist put it, "empirical work is deeply infused with theory: empirical researchers do not discover what 'is,' but rather—much like philosophers—they make an argument about the social world in dialectical relationships with existing theory."[58] This influence explains why, for example, the same empirical findings can be interpreted differently by people with different substantive views on the ethical issues under consideration.[59]

Qualitative research can help with this problem. Qualitative studies present open-ended questions that give subjects freedom to bring up their own concerns. As a result, such studies are more likely to elicit subjects' independent viewpoints than are forced-choice surveys and questionnaires. Once obtained, qualitative data can be used to develop surveys and questionnaires that take into account subjects' own ideas about the research experience. Including experienced subjects in study planning and data interpretation can also lead to more informative empirical studies of subject perspectives.

Subject narratives are another important information source. Previous chapters include a variety of published narratives describing what study participation was like for certain individuals. Narratives tend to convey a more vivid and detailed picture of the subject experience than empirical investigations do. Narratives are also accessible to just about everyone.[60] Subjects' stories give both experts and ordinary people a rich sense of what study participation can be like.

Of course, narratives have weaknesses too. Some experts dismiss the use of narrative evidence in ethics and policy deliberations, claiming that such evidence is unrepresentative and prone to inaccuracy. Chapter 6 describes problems that can arise when research policy decisions rely on unrepresentative samples of patient narratives. "Right to try" laws are an example of what can happen when officials respond to only one kind of patient narrative.

But bias and distortion are not inevitable in the use of subject narratives. In the medical arena, patient narratives play a major role in website and other evaluations of patient care. On the belief that "representative, fulsome, coherent accounts of patient experience" can enhance evaluations of medical care, policy analysts are developing a rigorous approach to the use of narrative evidence in that setting. Such an approach includes, for example, making affirmative efforts to gather narratives from large groups of patients rather than relying only on narratives that patients submit on their own initiative.[61] Similar strategies could be applied to strengthen the value of subject narratives in research decision-making.

Incorporating Subject Perspectives into Research Decisions

The effort to take subject perspectives into account will face additional challenges. One involves what has been labeled the "heterogeneity problem." The heterogeneity problem exists because like research professionals, experienced subjects have diverse views on research and research ethics. In many instances, empirical studies on subject perspectives are "not a path to greater universality, but to greater particularity."[62] Studies that uncover greater particularity call into question the application of rules and practices built on unitary assumptions about subject experiences.

The results of an interview study involving subjects of cancer genetics research illustrate the heterogeneity of subjects' views. For years, ethicists and other professionals have disagreed on the best model for the relationship between researchers and subjects. Should this relationship be more like the doctor-patient relationship, the legal contract relationship, the gift-giving relationship, or something else? On the belief that subjects' "views of the researcher-participant relationship are of equal importance to those of researchers, IRB professionals, and ethicists," one research team decided to study subjects' views.[63] The team found that subjects had complicated views about the researcher-subject relationship, with most describing features of more than one model.

Some subjects saw the relationship as collaborative, but not necessarily egalitarian. More than half thought the relationship shared elements of the doctor-patient relationship. Subjects in this group expected to be informed of any study findings that could have personal health consequences for them. At the same time, most subjects wanted a less intense relationship with researchers than they had with physicians. The majority preferred a "limited, professional, but cordial" relationship with researchers.[64] These results offer useful information, but they show that participants' perspectives are neither simple nor uniform.

Findings like these complicate efforts to create general rules and guidelines reflecting subject perspectives. It isn't always easy to capture subject perspectives in a single rule or guideline. When subjects hold diverse views, which of those views should rules and guidelines take into account? In such situations, there is a potential "tyranny of the majority."[65] Should the majority prevail, or should minority views also be respected?

A second study puts the latter questions into stark relief. In this study, investigators distributed a survey asking 1,095 adults whether they thought consent should be required in three hypothetical trials evaluating standard medical practices. About half the survey respondents thought that subjects' written permission should be required to conduct the trials. About one-quarter said that verbal consent would be acceptable. The survey then asked respondents what they would prefer if the logistics of asking patients for written or verbal consent made it too difficult to conduct the trials. Although many said it would be acceptable to dispense with consent requirements in those circumstances, about one-third said the research should not be conducted without written or oral consent.[66]

As the survey team noted, a central question raised by their findings is whether research rules should be designed to favor the "consent-requiring minority" or the "research-supporting majority." The informed consent requirement is intended to protect an individual's freedom to decide on research participation. Would it be defensible to ignore the substantial minority position and dispense with consent requirements? Or should the minority position determine policy, because a failure to require consent would severely restrict individual liberty?[67]

A related challenge is determining the degree of influence subject preferences should have on research ethics and policy decisions. Experienced subjects are one of many groups with a legitimate interest in such decisions. What should happen when subjects' views on an issue differ from those of other stakeholders, such as researchers, ethicists, patient advocates, and members of the general public? What weight should subjects' views have relative to the views of others participating in research decision-making?

The proper answers to these questions will depend on the task at hand. In some situations, it would be reasonable and justifiable to give subjects' views relatively substantial weight. For example, if a majority of experienced subjects advising an IRB believed that it would be wrong for researchers to withhold certain study information from prospective subjects, the subjects' position should prevail. In this situation, experienced subjects would be most qualified to decide what information a reasonable person would want to know about the study.

In other situations, the views of experienced subjects could tip the balance in favor of a particular decision. Such an approach would be justified, for example, when members of an advisory group agree that two or more policy options would be acceptable. The distinct value of knowledge gained through personal research experience would be a reason to make subjects' views the determining factor in such a case.

Developing a subject inclusion program will require planners to attend to all of these challenges. As one team commented, "studying and integrating participants' perspectives into research ethics would be easier if participants' views were simple, homogeneous, and stable."[68] Yet the data reveal a more complex picture. This complexity makes it more challenging to include subjects' perspectives, but the challenges are far from insurmountable. The complex perspectives of researchers, ethicists, and members of the public are reflected in research ethics and policy, and subjects' complex perspectives should be added to the mix.

FROM RHETORIC TO REALITY

Talk of patients and subjects as research partners has never been more popular than it is today. Officials leading projects like the NIH Precision Medicine Initiative say they want to change rules and practices to bring them "more in line with participants' desire to be active partners in modern science."[69] Experts recognize the need for "new norms and mechanisms" to govern the growing practice of subject-led research—norms and mechanisms that give participants more power than is customary in traditional research.[70] In the new research environment, these experts say, "the boundary between researcher and subject will blur, with important consequences for the way we think about research regulation and research ethics."[71]

Yet the subjects-as-partners rhetoric is nothing new. And for years, we have seen little effort to put these words into practice. If today's researchers, ethicists, and policy officials are serious about adopting a more egalitarian model, they will turn to experienced study subjects for help. Experienced subjects have knowledge that qualifies them to be real research collaborators.

There are some signs of progress in creating true partnerships. Engaging communities and developing patient-centered models of human research are moves in the right direction. But experts should recognize the distinct contribution that experienced subjects can make to such efforts. Research ethicists and policy officials should adopt a more inclusive approach too. It's time for everyone to learn what subjects can teach about the ethics of human research.

NOTES

1. Alexander Capron, "Subjects, Participants, and Partners: What Are the Implications for Research as the Role of Informed Consent Evolves?," in *Human Subjects Research Regulation: Perspectives on the Future*, ed. I. Glenn Cohen and Holly Fernandez Lynch (Cambridge, MA: MIT Press, 2014), 154–68, 162.
2. Michael McDonald, Susan Cox, and Anne Townsend, "Toward Human Research Protection That Is Evidence Based and Participant Centered," in Cohen and Lynch, *Human Subjects Research Regulation*, 124–38, 134. These analysts regard the current exclusion of subjects from research decision-making as similar to the exclusionary practices that gave rise to the disability rights movement. They believe the disability movement slogan, "Nothing about us without us," applies to research participants as well. Ibid., 132.
3. Rhonda Kost et al., "Assessing Research Participants' Perceptions of Their Research Experiences," *Clinical and Translational Science* 4 (2011): 403–13, 409.
4. Nancy Campbell and Laura Stark, "Making Up 'Vulnerable' People: Human Subjects and the Subjective Experience of Medical Experiment," *Social History of Medicine* 28 (2015): 825–48.
5. Ibid., 846.
6. Ibid., 829.
7. Celia Fisher, "Ethics in Drug Abuse and Related HIV Risk Research," *Applied Developmental Science* 8 (2004): 91–103, 92.
8. Celia Fisher, "A Relational Perspective on Ethics-in-Science Decisionmaking for Research with Vulnerable Populations," *IRB: A Review of Human Subjects Research* 19, no. 5 (1997): 1–4, 2.
9. Joint United Nations Programme on HIV/AIDS, *Good Participatory Practice: Guidelines for Biomedical HIV Prevention Trials*, 2nd ed., 2011. Retrieved November 18, 2015, from http://www.avac.org/resource/good-participatory-practice-guidelines-biomedical-hiv-prevention-trials-second-edition-0.
10. "Federal Policy for the Protection of Human Subjects," 56 *Fed. Reg.* 28014 (June 18, 1991).

11. For example, one unaffiliated member wrote, "I do try to represent, advocate for, and guard the rights of the potential study participant." Marcia Slaven, "First Impressions: The Experiences of a Community Member on a Research Ethics Committee," *IRB: Ethics & Human Research* 29, no. 3 (2007): 17–19, 18. In one survey, 83 percent of nonscientist and unaffiliated IRB members saw their role as being an advocate for human subjects. Joan Porter, "How Unaffiliated/ Nonscientist Members of Institutional Review Boards See Their Roles," *IRB: A Review of Human Subject Research* 9, no. 6 (1987): 1–6.

12. Charles Lidz et al., "The Participation of Community Members on Medical IRBs," *Journal of Empirical Research on Human Research Ethics* 7, no. 1 (2012): 1–8, 6.

13. Sohini Sengupta and Bernard Lo, "The Role and Experiences of Nonaffiliated and Non-scientist Members of Institutional Review Boards," *Academic Medicine* 78 (2003): 212–18.

14. As Laura Stark has observed, the regulations "require [experts] to imagine the perspectives of people whom the law is controlling or safeguarding." Laura Stark, *Behind Closed Doors: IRBs and the Making of Ethical Research* (Chicago: University of Chicago Press, 2012), 13.

15. Ann Cook, Helena Hoas, and Jane Joyner, "The Protector and the Protected: What Regulators and Researchers Can Learn from IRB Members and Subjects," *Narrative Inquiry in Bioethics* 3 (2013): 51–65, 60.

16. Emily Anderson, "A Qualitative Study of Non-affiliated, Non-scientist Institutional Review Board Members," *Accountability in Research* 13 (2006): 135–51. There are exceptions, however. One unaffiliated member wrote that for a few people like her, "the motivation to serve is more personal. We or our loved ones have been research subjects, so we bear an especially poignant responsibility. The memory of the peculiarly uneven power relationship between investigator and subject is one that still burns bright." Patricia Bauer, "A Few Simple Truths about Your Community Members," *IRB: Ethics & Human Research* 23, no. 1 (2001): 7–8.

17. Stark, *Behind Closed Doors*, 14–15.

18. Institute of Medicine Committee on Assessing the System for Protecting Human Research Subjects, *Preserving Public Trust: Accreditation and Human Research Participant Protection Programs* (Washington, DC: National Academies Press, 2001), 73 & note 3. A report from President Bill Clinton's bioethics advisory group said that IRBs should include members who "reflect the views of the research participants." National Bioethics Advisory Commission, *Ethical and Policy Issues in Research Involving Human Participants* (2001), 63. Retrieved April 21, 2015, from https://bioethicsarchive.georgetown.edu/nbac/human/overvol1.pdf.

19. Association for the Accreditation of Human Research Protection Programs, "Domain II: Institutional Review Board or Ethics Committee" (2009). Retrieved April 20, 2015, from http://www.aahrpp.org/apply/web-document-library/domain-ii-institutional-review-board-or-ethics-committee.

20. Marjorie Speers and Susan Rose, "Labeling Institutional Review Board Members Does Not Lead to Better Protections for Research Participants," *Academic Medicine* 87 (2012): 842–44. For similar arguments, see McDonald, Cox, and Townsend, "Toward Human Research Protection"; Govind Persad, "Democratic Deliberation and the Ethical Review of Human Subject Research," in Cohen and Lynch, *Human Subjects Research Regulation*, 169–84; Duke Morrow, "Missing Subjects," *IRB: Ethics & Human Research* 30, no. 4 (2008): 19–20.

21. Jonathan Moreno, *Undue Risk: Secret State Experiments on Humans* (New York: W. H. Freeman, 2000), 281.

22. Institute of Medicine Committee, *Preserving Public Trust*, 8. Others argue that the human research oversight system should actively track subjects' experiences in trials. The current system relies largely on subject- and researcher-initiated reports for information about potential problems in ongoing studies. McDonald, Cox, and Townsend, "Toward Human Research Protection," 131.

23. Existing US research regulations permit IRBs to consult "individuals with competence in special areas" about issues that require particular expertise. "Federal Policy for the Protection of Human Subjects," 28,015. Experienced subjects

are "experiential experts" who could be asked to weigh in on relevant issues. See Persad, "Democratic Deliberation," 178.

24. One research team has developed a standardized survey to assess subjects' perceptions. See Rhonda Kost et al., "Assessing Participant-Centered Outcomes to Improve Clinical Research," *New England Journal of Medicine* 369 (2013): 2179–81.

25. See External Review of Human Research Protections, University of Minnesota, Final Report (February 25, 2015). Retrieved December 1, 2015, from http://research.umn.edu/advancehrp/external-review.html.

26. For description and discussion of these models, see Rebecca Dresser, *When Science Offers Salvation: Patient Advocacy and Research Ethics* (New York: Oxford University Press, 2001), 21–43; Adam Braddock, "Children as Research Partners in Community Pediatrics," in Cohen and Lynch, *Human Subjects Research Regulation*, 93–105; Juan Domecq et al., "Patient Engagement in Research: A Systematic Review," *BMC Health Services Research* 14 (2014): 89–98; Joseph Selby, Laura Forsythe, and Harold Sox, "Stakeholder-Driven Comparative Research: An Update from PCORI," *Journal of the American Medical Association* 314 (2015): 2235–36; Raymond De Vries et al., "Assessing the Quality of Democratic Deliberation: A Case Study of Public Deliberation on the Ethics of Surrogate Consent for Research," *Social Science and Medicine* 70 (2010): 1896–903; Loretta Jones and Kenneth Wells, "Strategies for Academic and Clinician Engagement in Community-Participatory Partnered Research," *Journal of the American Medical Association* 297 (2007): 407–8.

27. See Domecq et al., "Patient Engagement," 89.

28. See Dresser, *When Science Offers Salvation*, 28–29, 32–33. See also Lois Frank et al., "The PCORI Perspective on Patient-Centered Outcomes Research," *Journal of the American Medical Association*, 312 (2014): 1513–14, which notes that "Patients have unique perspectives that can change and improve the pursuit of clinical [research] questions."

29. National Institutes of Health Clinical and Translational Science Awards Consortium, *Principles of Community*

Engagement, 2nd ed. (2011). Retrieved April 21, 2015, from www.atsdr.cdc.gov/communityengagement/.

30. Shawn Kneipp et al., "Women's Experiences in a Community-Based Participatory Research Randomized Controlled Trial," *Qualitative Health Research* 23 (2013): 847–60, 856.

31. Domecq et al., "Patient Engagement," 89. See also Dresser, *When Science Offers Salvation*, 29–32.

32. Julie Brintnall-Karabelas et al., "Improving Recruitment in Clinical Trials: Why Eligible Participants Decline," *Journal of Empirical Research on Human Research Ethics* 6, no. 1 (2011): 69–74, 71; Patrina Caldwell et al., "Parents' Attitudes toward Children's Participation in Randomized Controlled Trials," *Journal of Pediatrics* 142 (2003): 554–59.

33. See Patricia Marshall et al., "Negotiating Decisions during Informed Consent for Pediatric Phase I Oncology Trials," *Journal of Empirical Research on Human Research Ethics* 7, no. 2 (2012): 51–59, which describes negotiations on such matters between researchers and parents of children in cancer trials. Another research group urged other researchers to "recognize the immense responsibility that proxy decision makers must shoulder, not only ethically but also physically, emotionally, and logistically" and to offer services such as transportation as part of a study protocol. Laura Dunn et al., "'Thinking about It for Somebody Else': Alzheimer's Disease Research and Proxy Decision Makers' Translation of Ethical Principles into Practice," *American Journal of Geriatric Psychiatry* 21 (2013): 337–45, 344.

34. See C. Daniel Mullins et al., "Patient Centeredness in the Design of Clinical Trials," *Value in Health* 17 (2014): 471–76; Peter Korn, "Clinical Trials Stymied as Patients Balk at 'Experiments,'" *Portland Tribune*, January 16, 2014. Retrieved April 15, 2015, from http://portlandtribune.com/pt/9-news/207447-63461-clinical-trials-stymied-as-patients-balk-at-experiments.

35. See Mullins et al., "Patient Centeredness," which describes such methods.

36. See Emily Anderson, "Learning from Research Participants," *American Journal of Bioethics* 15, no. 11 (2015): 14–16.

37. Sandra Quinn et al., "Improving Informed Consent with Minority Participants: Results from Researcher and

Community Surveys," *Journal of Empirical Research on Human Subject Research* 7, no. 4 (2012): 44–55, 49. Another research group reported that parents of children in cancer trials sought support through speaking with parents of children who had already experienced the research decision-making process. Michelle Eder et al., "Improving Informed Consent: Suggestions from Parents of Children with Leukemia," *Pediatrics* 119 (2007): e849–59, e855.

38. Yoram Unguro, Anne Sill, and Naynesh Kamini, "Experiences of Children Enrolled in Pediatric Oncology Research: Implications for Assent," *Pediatrics* 125 (2010): e876–83, e880.

39. C. Behrendt et al., "What Do Our Patients Understand about Their Trial Participation? Assessing Patients' Understanding of Their Informed Consent Consultation about Randomized Clinical Trials," *Journal of Medical Ethics* 37 (2011): 74–80, 78.

40. Eric Kodish et al., "Communication of Randomization in Childhood Leukemia Trials," *Journal of the American Medical Association* 291 (2004): 470–75, 474.

41. For proposals to this effect, see Rebecca Dresser, "Aligning Regulations and Ethics in Human Research," *Science* 337 (2012): 527–28; David Wendler, "Can We Ensure That All Subjects Give Valid Consent?," *Archives of Internal Medicine* 164 (2004): 2201–4. In one study, parents of children in cancer trials told interviewers that the decision process should include more breaks to check on parents' understanding and allow them to ask questions. Eder et al., "Improving Informed Consent," e858.

42. See, for example, Ruth Faden et al., "An Ethics Framework for a Learning Health Care System: A Departure from Traditional Research Ethics and Clinical Ethics," *Hastings Center Report* 43, no. 1 (2013): S16–27.

43. Ibid., S23.

44. See, for example, Jerry Menikoff, "The Unbearable Rightness of Being in Clinical Trials," *Hastings Center Report* 43, no. 1 (2013): S30–31.

45. See Jeremy Sugarman and Robert Califf, "Ethics and Regulatory Complexities for Pragmatic Clinical Trials," *Journal of the American Medical Association* 311 (2014): 2381–82.

46. For an argument that researchers should rely on a community engagement process to determine what a reasonable participant would want to know about a study, see Emily Anderson and Stephanie Solomon, "Community Engagement: Critical to Continued Public Trust in Research," *American Journal of Bioethics* 13, no. 12 (2013): 44–46. For an argument that a group of ordinary people, rather than an IRB composed primarily of health professionals, should decide when full consent is required, see Rebecca Dresser, "Is Informed Consent Always Necessary for Randomized Clinical Trials?," *New England Journal of Medicine* 341 (1999): 448.

47. For discussion on involving participants in the development of best practices for research, see Susan Cox and Michael MacDonald, "Ethics Is for Human Subjects Too: Participant Perspectives on Responsibility in Health Research," *Social Science and Medicine* 98 (2013): 224–31.

48. For discussion of advertising and recruitment, see David Hunter, "We Could Be Heroes: Ethical Issues with the Pre-recruitment of Research Participants," *Journal of Medical Ethics* 41 (2015): 557–58. For discussion of subject responsibilities and risk limits, see David Resnik and Elizabeth Ness, "Participants' Responsibilities in Clinical Research," *Journal of Medical Ethics* 38 (2011): 746–50; Sarah Edwards, "Assessing the Remedy: The Case for Contracts in Clinical Trials," *American Journal of Bioethics* 11, no. 4 (2011): 3–12; Franklin Miller and Steven Joffe, "Limits to Research Risks," *Journal of Medical Ethics* 35 (2009): 445–49.

49. See Dresser, *When Science Offers Salvation*, 109–28.

50. Elizabeth Bromley et al., "From Subject to Participant: Ethics and the Evolving Role of Community in Health Research," *American Journal of Public Health* 105 (2015): 900–908; Mark Schlesinger et al., "Taking Patients' Narratives about Clinicians from Anecdotes to Science," *New England Journal of Medicine* 373 (2015): 675–79.

51. Paul Lombardo, "New Faces on the IRB: Who Speaks for Subjects?," special section, *BioLaw* (September–October 1999): S428–31.

52. See Lisa Mikesell, Elizabeth Bromley, and Dmitry Khodyakov, "Ethical Community-Engaged Research: A Literature

Review," *American Journal of Public Health* 103 (2013): e7–13; Rachael Fleurence et al., "Engaging Patients and Stakeholders in Research Proposal Review: The Patient-Centered Outcomes Research Institute," *Annals of Internal Medicine* 161 (2014): 122–30.

53. Antoine Boiven et al., "What Are the Key Ingredients for Effective Public Involvement in Health Care Improvement and Policy Decisions? A Randomized Trial Process Evaluation," *Milbank Quarterly* 92 (2014): 319–50.

54. Ibid., 333.

55. For example, the UNAIDS guidelines for participatory research portray education as essential to producing the "research literacy" that enables community participants to make meaningful contributions to research activities. Joint United Nations Programme, *Good Participatory Practice*, 20, 36–38. The Patient-Centered Outcomes Research Institute has called for more studies comparing approaches to engaging stakeholders with diverse perspectives and integrating those perspectives into peer review. Fleurence et al., "Engaging Patients and Stakeholders," 129.

56. See Dresser, *When Science Offers Salvation*, 121–43; Steven Epstein, *Impure Science: AIDS, Activism, and the Politics of Knowledge* (Berkeley: University of California Press, 1996), 337–46.

57. For example, the Research Advocacy Network provides educational materials and workshops for lay advocates (researchadvocacy.org), as does the National Breast Cancer Coalition through its Project LEAD (breastcancerdeadline2020.org).

58. Stacy Carter, "Beware Dichotomies and Grand Abstractions: Attending to Particularity and Practice in Empirical Bioethics," *American Journal of Bioethics* 9, no. 6–7 (2009): 76–77.

59. For example, ethicists presented different interpretations of empirical data from a public survey on attitudes toward informed consent in three hypothetical studies. Some ethicists thought the survey responses supported allowing the studies to be conducted without consent if seeking consent would be logistically difficult. Others thought the responses showed

that most people would want to be notified about the studies and that most preferred a requirement for some form of individual consent. See Mildred Cho et al., "Attitudes toward Risk and Informed Consent for Research on Medical Practices," *Annals of Internal Medicine* 162 (2015): 690–96; John Lantos, "U.S. Research Regulations: Do They Reflect the Views of the People They Claim to Protect?," *Annals of Internal Medicine* 162 (2015): 731–32; Lois Shepherd et al., "Comment," *Annals of Internal Medicine* 162 (2015): 725–26.

60. See Louise Aronson, "Story as Evidence, Evidence as Story," *Journal of the American Medical Association* 314 (2015): 125–26.

61. Schlesinger et al., "Taking Patients' Narratives."

62. Carter, "Beware Dichotomies and Grand Abstractions," 77.

63. Celeste Condit et al., "What Should Be the Character of the Researcher-Participant Relationship?," *IRB: Ethics & Human Research* 37, no. 4 (2015): 1–10, 2.

64. Ibid., 8.

65. Celia Fisher, "Relational Perspective," 3.

66. Cho et al., "Attitudes toward Risk."

67. For discussion of aggregation issues related to risk-benefit assessments, see Michelle Meyer, "Three Challenges for Risk-Based (Research) Regulation: Heterogeneity among Regulated Activities, Regulator Bias, and Stakeholder Heterogeneity," in Cohen and Lynch, *Human Subjects Research Regulation*, 323–37.

68. Condit et al., "What Should Be the Character," 9. Celia Fisher was not surprised when her interview study found diversity in street-drug users' views of ethical issues in addiction research. Fisher commented that just as "[s]cientists and IRBs do not expect nondeliberative, categorical, or decontextualized answers from their colleagues on such complex issues," they should not expect such answers from members of the research population. Celia Fisher, "Addiction Research Ethics and the Belmont Principles: Do Drug Users Have a Different Moral Voice?," *Substance Use & Misuse* 46 (2011): 728–41, 738.

69. Francis Collins and Harold Varmus, "A New Initiative on Precision Medicine," *New England Journal of Medicine* 372 (2015): 793–95.

70. Effy Vayena et al., "Research Led by Participants: A New Social Contract for a New Kind of Research," *Journal of Medical Ethics*. Published online first: April 13, 2015, doi:10.1136/medethics-2015-102663.

71. Dan O'Connor, "The Apomediated World: Regulating Research When Social Media Has Changed Research," *Journal of Law, Medicine & Ethics* 41 (2013): 470–83, 472.

INDEX

Printed in the USA/Agawam, MA
December 29, 2017

666397.002